Table of Contents

Introduction 5

Chapter 1: Why Hormones Matter 13

Chapter 2: The Gift of Surrogacy 23

Chapter 3: Giving Grace.. 34

Chapter 4: Hormones, Chemical Exposure, and You 43

Chapter 5: Hormones and Your Physical Health 48

Chapter 6: Hormones and Your Mental Health 65

Chapter 7: Hormones and Sexual Health 79

Chapter 8: Simple Swaps 93

Chapter 9: Moving Forward 115

About the Authors 117

Photos 118

References 123

Introduction

Have you ever struggled with something in your life that nearly broke you? Had a health issue that consumed you and took over your life? Suffered from something, diagnosed or undiagnosed, without any explanation as to why it occurred? A condition that brought out every insecurity you've ever had? Confronted you with everything you've been afraid of and turned you into someone you didn't recognize? Something that caused you to challenge and start doubting everything you've dreamed of, so much so that you felt hopeless, depressed, and worthless?

I did...we did.

For 14 years, my husband, Ben, and I struggled with unexplained infertility–something that nearly ruined me...and us. I pushed away people I loved and changed my social circles because it was too difficult to see the people I loved live the dream I so desperately wanted. The body I worked so hard to take care of-eating healthy, exercising daily, taking supplements, meeting with countless doctors, therapists, nutritionists, acupuncturists-all without results. Month after month, year after year, constantly feeling like a failure.

Our diagnosis of "unexplained infertility" didn't cut it; I wanted the doctors to find something wrong and fix it. The only relief we found with our unexplained infertility diagnosis was when any uneducated and insensitive person inquiring about our fertility struggle would ask, "Whose fault is it?" We would respond that it was unexplained. Infertility isn't ever anyone's "fault."

During our 6th round of IVF, I broke down at our doctor's office. We were working with one of the best doctors in the world, we had altered our lifestyle and diets significantly, and each round of IVF was not only incredibly expensive but also physically and mentally exhausting. It took a huge toll on my mental health, and was difficult on our relationship as well. We didn't know how much more we could do.

We asked our doctor if there was anything else we could do to improve our chances of conceiving. What he told us that day changed our lives forever. He asked what skincare, home care, and wellness products we were using, sharing that there were chemicals in these products that could impact our hormones. We were shocked, although as we thought more about it, it made complete sense.

With each round of IVF, the doctors would monitor my hormones closely. I was prescribed a hormone cream–I would apply a small amount on my skin at night and go to the doctor the next morning to get my blood levels tested. By morning, my bloodwork showed a dramatic hormone spike. How hadn't we put two and two together earlier? If that tiny amount of cream could affect my hormones in such a significant way, other products we were putting on our bodies could as well.

If you think about the nicotine or pain patch, you apply a patch on your skin, its contents get into your bloodstream, and you can feel the effects almost immediately. If a patch had such an influence on how our bodies performed, other products could as well. We didn't know why we hadn't fully realized earlier that the products we were putting **on, in, and around** our bodies could impact our hormones, positively or negatively.

With this new knowledge, we dove into the research. We learned that we are exposed to dozens of harmful chemicals every day from products that we use, and hundreds more from the chemicals in our homes and environment. These chemicals impact our hormones and can lead to significant physical, mental, and sexual health issues and diseases. How could we help create solutions that would help limit our chemical exposure?

During our infertility struggle, Ben and I were incredibly private; it was too painful to discuss, and we didn't want to answer questions month after month with each failed attempt. We didn't tell close friends or even our families that we were trying. It wasn't until ten years into our struggle, when I finally shared our news with my sister-in-law, that our lives completely changed. She incredibly volunteered to be our gestational surrogate and carried our son, Hugh. When Hugh was almost one, my sister called and volunteered to be our second surrogate, and gave birth to our daughter, Grace. Both offers were a complete surprise, and we learned a valuable lesson: vulnerability is a strength, and sometimes it can create miracles. We'll share many more personal details about our surrogacy experience throughout this book.

We finally had our Hugh and our Grace; our family was complete. We couldn't believe how fortunate we were; we thankfully had great careers which helped us afford all our medical procedures along the way, and now we had our two little miracles. Everything seemed to be perfect.

But after having Grace, I couldn't sleep at night, but not because we had a crying newborn. So many people made huge sacrifices to help us have our miracles, and what we learned about hormone health impacts everyone. I felt a huge responsibility to pay forward the generosity we had received.

When we initially learned about hormone disruption and hormone health, we had only associated the role of hormones with fertility, given that it was our entire focus for 14 years. As we started diving deeper into the research and data, we learned hormone disruption impacted way more than just infertility…it is associated with many other health issues, including depression, anxiety, autoimmune diseases, obesity, cancers, and many more headline diseases. Hormone disruption's annual cost in the US is hundreds of billions of dollars. Hormone disruption impacts <u>everyone.</u>

Knowing the damage that hormone disruption has on our health, we started researching hormone health benefits, which include reduced stress levels, restful sleep, clear skin, weight management, gut health, and longevity; benefits all of us want. How could we help build awareness around this topic while also providing real solutions that were simple, elevated, and effective, and also promoted hormone health?

Clearly, no single product or product line could fully address this topic; it needed to be a lifestyle approach. We also needed to create more than just products—a comprehensive holistic solution meant creating awareness, education and community, along with products. If we could educate consumers on how to make simple, daily swaps to help promote hormone health and reduce their exposure to harmful chemicals, we could empower them to support their physical, mental, and sexual health, and live simpler, healthier and happier lives.

We knew what we needed to create…we weren't sure how exactly we would do it with a newborn and a barely 2-year-old. What we did know was that we couldn't not start this business.

After having Hugh and Grace, Ben and I seriously considered what kind of lives we wanted to live. What did success look like to us personally? We both had great careers that we enjoyed. Ben managed a billion dollar family office in Beverly Hills, overseeing global investments and operating businesses. I spent my career in philanthropy, developing relationships with executives and thought leaders, raising tens of millions for nonprofits and higher education, helping them create legacy gifts with meaningful donations. We both have master's degrees from the University of Southern California, and I enjoyed working on the major gifts team for USC Marshall.

While we loved and enjoyed our careers, Ben worked long and late hours, and I was constantly traveling. We finally had our littles, and it felt like a cloud was lifted–we saw our lives in a new light. We wanted to live differently: we wanted to spend time with our kiddos, share the knowledge we had learned, and create an impact. So, when Grace was a newborn and Hugh was barely two years old, we decided to launch our business. It was one of the scariest times in our lives.

We both resigned from our careers (I resigned during my maternity leave with Grace; I never received maternity leave for Hugh, but that's for another story) and started our business. What better name for our company could there be than for the very purpose our company was founded, we named our company Hugh & Grace. The name Hugh means heart, mind and spirit, and Grace means goodness, generosity and love. Those are the qualities that helped bring us our miracles, and also our company values.

Our mission is to promote hormone health and help reduce harmful chemical exposure through high-performance products, trusted education, and an inclusive community. We knew what we needed to create and were excited to launch our company, but launching just as a global health crisis unfolded quickly turned our excitement into intensity, uncertainty, and fear. That time was one of the scariest and most stressful times in our lives. Due to Covid, our investors pulled out, and we were forced to invest all of our liquidity and leave all our financial security as we poured everything we had into something we hoped and believed could truly change the world.

Ben and I are fortunate to have incredible professional and personal networks and could get an introduction to almost anyone. How could we leverage our relationships for good? We began making calls, asking for introductions to top formulators, manufacturers, and experts across various fields and product categories. We assembled our medical advisory board, including world-renowned doctors and hormone health experts. We flew across the country, meeting with CEOs and innovation teams of some of the largest and most respected formulators in the world. During those early months and years, we dedicated ourselves to formulating, testing, and refining high-performance, hormone supportive products that add real value–products that are versatile, good for men, women and kids. Despite nearly a year of delays due to COVID-19 restrictions, we successfully launched Hugh & Grace on May 22, 2021, and have been working nonstop ever since.

Over the years, I've been asked how I had the confidence to give up all of our security with such a young family and create our company, investing every dollar we had without knowing if it would be successful. While I've had many fantastic people in my life who have loved and supported me, I give the most credit to Ben, who has always believed in me, even during all the years when I didn't believe in myself. You'll learn more throughout this book about how incredible Ben is.

Another role model who profoundly shaped my life was my grandfather, Dale Tingey. He founded American Indian Services (AIS), one of the nation's longest-running American Indian scholarship organizations, providing both scholarships and employment opportunities to Native Americans.

Every summer, we visited my grandparents. As the oldest grandchild, I had the privilege of joining my grandfather on his work trips to Native American reservations across the West. A World War II pilot, he owned a small Cessna and would fly us from one reservation to the next, often staying for days at a time to better understand each tribe's needs. When I was little, we delivered donated goods, and I spent my days playing with the children and learning traditional dances. As I grew older, he invited me to speak at events and attend meetings with chiefs and Navajo Nation leaders. I volunteered at fundraising events, joined donor meetings, and traveled the world with him. I witnessed firsthand how communities were impacted when someone genuinely cared and took action.

My grandfather was humble and rarely spoke about himself. Over the course of his career, he worked with U.S. Presidents, top executives, professional athletes, and celebrities. He gave everything he had and never hesitated to ask for help if it meant advancing an important cause. The running joke was that he would always give the shirt off his back to help someone - and the shirts off all his friends' backs as well.

He passed away at the age of 100. Even in his final years, when he was bedridden, he continued to make an impact, raising funds by making calls from his bed. He was my hero. He showed me that when people come together around an important mission, lives are transformed and miracles happen.

With Hugh & Grace, it was time for Ben and me to give the shirts off our backs…and ask our friends for the shirts off their friends' backs as well. In the past few years, we've made thousands of calls to our friends, experts and doctors asking for help, intros, or investments. If any of our friends are reading this, we are so appreciative of your support. We even called in favors for this book from several world-renowned experts who are thought leaders in their fields and who have become close friends. They have contributed their knowledge about the important role hormones play in our physical, mental, and sexual health. In this book, Ben and I, along with this collection of friends, changemakers, and experts, will share our personal experiences and learnings about hormone health. We'll also share how, by making daily simple swaps, you can also make a significant impact on your overall health and well-being.

Ben and I wrote this book not to share our story but to provide you with actionable, simple tips and learnings that we gained throughout our journey; information we would have given anything to have during our struggle. Information that could have possibly helped avoid much of the trauma we went through. Our goal is to provide you with hope and resources that can help you live a simpler, healthier, and happier life.

Sara

CHAPTER 1

Why Hormones Matter

What were we thinking?? Just as we were preparing to launch our business, COVID hit, and every investor we had lined up pulled out. We were at a crossroads: should we continue or give up on our dream entirely? We had spent over a decade learning about hormone health in very real and personal ways, and after having our miracle children via surrogacy, we felt a deep responsibility to pay forward the generosity we received. We had learned that hormone health impacts everyone, and that hormone imbalances can lead to devastating health issues, including cancers, infertility and mental health diseases. We had set out to create far more than just a business; we envisioned a holistic preventative wellness solution which included creating awareness, knowledge and community, paired with high-performance, hormone supportive products.

We had left behind successful careers that we loved and took a huge risk in starting our business. Grace was a newborn, and Hugh was barely two years old, so life was already busy with our littles, but we were also living through the most serious health crises in history and locked down in our home in Los Angeles. It took more grit than we knew we had and nearly every penny of our savings to get our company, Hugh & Grace, off the ground. We had just hired our first two employees right before COVID hit, and we stopped paying ourselves entirely to make sure we could pay our new team members. Our stress levels were at an all-time high, but we believed what we were creating would benefit everyone. It took countless sleepless nights, tears, and all our determination to create Hugh & Grace, and we did it all for this mission:

To empower you to live a simpler, healthier, happier life through improving your hormone health.

Everyone's busy. We're constantly racing from one thing to the next, rarely taking time to stop and think about how our everyday decisions impact our health. Hormone health has only recently started to be discussed, and there's a constant stream of information being shared. It can be difficult to decipher what information is accurate or how we activate that information to make decisions that are best for us and those we love. That is the "why" behind this book, and we aim to provide clear, actionable insights to help you make informed choices for a healthier life.

Hormones are chemical messengers in our bodies that regulate everything from our metabolism and sleep to our moods, libido, and even energy levels. When our hormones are in sync (the medical term is "homeostasis"), we look and feel great. But when our hormones are disrupted, so is our overall well-being, which can lead to serious physical, mental and sexual health issues.

From the outside looking in, we were "healthy." Ben was doing CrossFit, and I was an ultramarathoner. We ate healthy, exercised, and did everything "right" while trying to get pregnant, or so we thought. Unfortunately, we were never able to conceive, and what we learned from our doctors and research was that the topic of hormone health and hormone disruption is a massive topic that we felt compelled to address. Hormone-disrupting chemicals, also known as endocrine-disrupting chemicals (or EDCs), impact so much of our overall health. We knew that if we could create simple lifestyle solutions, hopefully others wouldn't have to experience the same struggles we had.

14 Years of Hell - by Sara

We married young; I was 23 and Ben was 26. We had dated for four years before getting married (long distance the last 2.5 years!). We got married the week after I graduated from college, moved to Vegas (Ben's hometown) and started our new lives together.

Growing up, I always wanted to be like my mom. She chose to be a stay-at-home mom (she left her career as a registered nurse in San Francisco after I was born) and invested all her time raising her five daughters and one son. My mother-in-law (who's also amazing) was a stay-at-home mom as well, raising her four sons and two daughters. Ben and I wanted a large family–we both agreed that four kids sounded like the perfect number for our family. I couldn't wait to be a stay-at-home mom.

Nothing could have prepared us for the next 14 years of our lives.

We began trying to get pregnant shortly after getting married…without success. Month after month, failed pregnancy test after failed pregnancy test, disappointment after disappointment. What were we doing wrong?? Supplements and ovulation strips didn't help. Sex (what was supposed to have been fun) soon became a chore, a reminder of our failure as we tried figuring out the best timing and position for the best chances of conception. The two-week wait to see if we were finally pregnant felt like an eternity, and then with each failed attempt, we'd have to wait another two weeks to try again. Cycle after cycle of hell.

We were young, doing everything "right" and were "healthy"…why wasn't it working?

"Are we doing this right?" I asked Ben.

We had just finished having sex, and I was lying on my back with pillows propped under my butt, my legs high in the air.

"I have to pee. Do I really have to stay like this for 20 minutes?"

"That's what Meghan said," Ben replied, tossing me a book to help distract me.

My legs were tingling, and my feet were starting to fall asleep, but I was determined to make sure I was doing everything possible. We had been trying to conceive for a few months, and I now hated the two-week waiting game almost as much as our negative pregnancy test results. Numb feet and legs would be worth it if it meant it worked this time.

Our friend Meghan had a hard time getting pregnant as well and had given us advice, but I was skeptical. I was peeing on ovulation strips daily and taking prenatal vitamins, but I didn't understand why I had to keep my feet in the air this long.

I was hesitant to ask my OB/GYN for advice. For some reason, I felt like that should be our last resort. Knowing how to get pregnant shouldn't be rocket science; we could surely figure out how to get pregnant without visiting a doctor. People had been making babies for centuries; it couldn't be that difficult. Until that point, sex had been fun and, from our perspective, pretty self-explanatory. We just assumed our bodies would work.

We were wrong.

So we started asking our doctor for help. And the next doctor. And the next specialist…and the next…and the next…and the next. We flew across the country and spent every dollar we made meeting with and learning from world-renowned experts in different medical fields: ob-gyns, urologists, pelvic floor specialists, endocrinologists, acupuncturists, therapists, hormone health and fertility experts.

For fourteen years.

And we never got pregnant.

When we were first trying to get pregnant, we knew very little about hormones besides the fact that we needed estrogen and testosterone to make a baby. Eventually, as we met with experts, we learned more. We spent countless hours in doctors' and specialists' offices, trying to figure out why we couldn't get pregnant, learning more and more about our bodies and hormones. It wasn't until much later that we learned how broad a topic hormone health is and how incredibly essential our hormones are to our overall health and well-being.

We sought out more and more specialists, traveling the country and meeting with experts, trying to figure out why we couldn't get pregnant. We were diagnosed with "unexplained infertility," a term physicians use to describe infertility after tests reveal no obvious cause for fertility struggles. The diagnosis is typically given only after both partners have undergone complete fertility evaluations and tests.

"Unexplained infertility is relatively frequent, affecting approximately 1 in 5 patients."
—Dr. Mark Surrey, M.D., F.A.C.O.G., F.A.C.S., and founder of Southern California Reproductive Center in Beverly Hills, CA.

However, with each appointment, the more we learned and the more questions we asked. Each appointment taught us more about how important hormones are to our overall health.

The first time we ever fully understood the direct impact of hormones on our health was during our sixth round of IVF. We were fortunate to be working with Dr. Mark Surrey, a world-renowned fertility doctor in Beverly Hills, and we were in deep conversation about what else we could be doing to improve our chances of conceiving. We had already changed our diets and lifestyles significantly. I loved to run and was an ultramarathoner, although I stopped running completely after hearing, "The running chicken doesn't lay good eggs." I hated needles, yet I went to acupuncture treatments three times a week. I couldn't take a job promotion because I needed to have flexibility in my work schedule to attend all my doctor, acupuncture and therapy visits.

Ben also made lifestyle changes. He enjoyed cycling, but stopped that as well. He avoided hot tubs at our doctor's recommendation to prevent any negative impact on his sperm production or motility. We were so desperate to have a baby that we were spending every dollar we made on therapy, doctors and medications. We were going crazy–what more could we do??

What Dr. Surrey shared with us next changed our lives forever.

"What skincare, homecare, and wellness products are you using? There are chemicals called hormone-disrupting chemicals or endocrine-disrupting chemicals (EDCs) in many of those products that are absorbed into your body and can disrupt your hormones."

During my IVF rounds, he was monitoring my hormones closely, and he had prescribed me a hormone cream as one of my medications. Each night, I would rub a small amount on my skin, and when I would get my blood levels tested the next morning, I would learn that my hormone levels had changed. If this small amount of cream could change my hormones, it made complete sense that other products could as well.

Understanding that the products we put **on, in, and around** us can impact our hormones, positively or negatively. We dove into the data and learned that the average American woman uses 12 products a day, unknowingly exposing herself to over 160 unique chemicals per day, and men to over 80 chemicals a day. We're also exposed to hundreds more in our environment.

The lifestyle changes we had been making had been so difficult, yet what Dr. Surrey shared seemed so simple. We were using expensive products from luxury brands; we had no clue that those products could negatively impact our hormones and contribute to our infertility.

We didn't know the extent of our exposure to harmful chemicals, just as we couldn't determine the exact cause of our inability to conceive. What we did know was that we needed to help create a solution to this growing, important problem.

Thankfully, as hormones are being discussed more, researchers have become more interested in the link between our bodies and our minds, specifically the role of hormones on our mental health. Hormones influence the production and regulation of neurotransmitters, which are chemicals that our brain cells use to communicate with each other. These neurotransmitters are essential for our mood regulation, sleep, focus, and overall well-being. Serotonin and dopamine are neurotransmitters known to impact happiness, motivation, and reward. When our hormone levels are imbalanced, neurotransmitter production can be affected, leading to symptoms of anxiety, depression, and other mental health conditions.

With each round of IVF, I was prescribed medications and injected hormones directly into my body, which not only impacted me physically with weight gain, bruising, and bloating but also severely impacted my moods and mental health. Looking back at everything we went through, we wish we had known how much hormones were linked to my mental health and mood swings instead of thinking I was literally going crazy.

I'm sharing one example below that, honestly, I'm not proud of, but I am sharing only to show the real impact hormones have on our mental health.

"Don't touch me!" I yelled, shoving Ben out of bed. "I stayed home trying to get pregnant all by myself while you were out with other women. Sleep in the guest bedroom!"

It was Tuesday at midnight, and Ben had just returned home from a work event, an LA Clippers game. We were nine days into my injections on our first round of IVF, and the hormones were definitely kicking in. Ben had made it his duty to give me every shot I needed and had never missed a day; he did it every morning and night. While undergoing IVF, I had strict limitations: I wasn't allowed to exercise, have sex, or drink caffeine or alcohol, that, combined with acupuncture, therapy, doctors' appointments, and blood work several times a week, was exhausting enough. I had canceled all my social plans for two weeks but didn't feel that both of our social lives should suffer. He offered to miss the game, but I had encouraged him to go, confident I would be ok. I gave myself the shot and went to bed early.

Ben hesitated, unsure of what had gone wrong. "There were women at the game, but I didn't talk to any. I was in a suite with all guys," he tried to reason with me.

I broke down in tears. I never cry! What were these hormone shots doing to me? Ben stood in the doorway, unsure whether he should go to the guest bedroom or try to console me; this was uncharted territory. I hadn't felt great on the shots, but up until now, it was manageable. I had done Clomid and IUI fertility treatments in the past, but I never experienced anything like this. This was PMS times a hundred.

We still had several more days of injections until our egg retrieval, when I would have to go under anesthesia for the procedure. The idea of me being passed out naked on an operating table and getting my eggs retrieved was not the way our pregnancy was supposed to happen. And we were paying nearly $30K for this pleasure?? This whole process was wrong.

If I knew then that I'd go through IVF 6 times without ever getting pregnant, I would have lost it then and there.

I knew I was a mess, and I felt terribly for Ben. During my hormone shots, I became a version of myself I couldn't recognize and began to hate. I was angry, emotional, and often irrational, all the while Ben remained calm and supportive. We were both hurting, yet Ben had to deal not only with the financial expense and disappointment of failed rounds of IVF but also with a crazy wife.

We've had several friends who immediately started undergoing fertility treatments after getting married for various reasons: some wanted the option to have multiple children, and some for age or health concerns. While we try never to give advice, we do share that we are so fortunate we had known each other for years before we underwent IVF. Ben knew me very well, so when I started acting crazy on my hormone shots, he knew it wasn't me, it was the hormones.

"Thankfully, I had known Sara for years before we started IVF, but there were still times I looked at the intensely emotional and volatile person she had become with a bit of fear, wondering if the woman I married was ever going to come back to me," Ben admits.

Honestly, I had the same concerns. I absolutely hated myself.

All of this was happening because of hormones, and our mental health was suffering.

The more Ben and I learned about our hormones and their impact on our bodies, physically and mentally, the more we started giving each other grace. I became more mindful of my mood changes during each cycle, and Ben knew when to give me space. Our hormones are so important to our overall health that after all of our fertility treatments, we both went to hormone therapy doctors to learn what we could do to improve our hormone health, which helped immensely. The more we learned, the greater we supported each other.

Over the years, Ben and I went to a lot of therapy, which was incredibly helpful in dealing with the high amount of stress and emotions we were experiencing. One of the most memorable experiences in my life was after one of our therapy sessions, about eight years into our fertility struggle. Earlier that week, we had learned our round of IVF had resulted in 0 healthy embryos. Saying we were devastated is an understatement. I was in my mid-thirties and overtly aware that my egg quality was declining with each passing year, which was adding pressure and even more stress. We had just left our therapy session, and I was emotionally exhausted. I didn't know how much more of this I could take.

Sensing my despair, Ben turned to me, put his hands around me and asked, "Sara, do we only want to be parents to our genetic children that you give birth to, or do we want to be parents? Because if we want to be parents, no matter what that looks like, we have time. "

I took a deep breath and felt a huge weight lift off my shoulders. I knew our answer. "Parents," I replied. He held me as I broke down sobbing, and we felt a whole new sense of hope. We could do this.

CHAPTER 2

The Gift of Surrogacy

The Conversation That Changed Our Lives – by Ben

The thought of not carrying our biological child had never occurred to us. We were so desperate to become parents and had already been through so much emotionally, physically, financially, and mentally that what happened next completely shocked Sara and me both. Before we dive in, I want to extend my deepest thanks to my stepsister, Jenna, and her family for their tremendous act of selflessness so that Sara and I could have the family we had always dreamed of.

Surrogacy completely changed our lives, and the resulting impact from our surrogacy experience has touched tens, if not hundreds, of thousands of others, directly or indirectly. We are incredibly fortunate to have two extraordinary women in our lives who didn't just agree to be our surrogates; they volunteered on their own without us even asking. This part of our life isn't always easy to talk about or even write about, but it is foundational to where we are today.

The first time we told anyone in our family about our fertility issues was in April of 2015, almost 10 years into our fertility struggle. My family had invited us to attend either a week-long family reunion or a day hike at the Grand Canyon. We had been pushing off seeing family for months because these events always reminded us of the lives we wanted but couldn't have. We knew we needed to see them, and a day hike would be the shortest option. So, we drove all night from LA to the Grand Canyon, arriving at the hotel way past midnight. We don't love hiking, and we started the day exhausted. We were dreading the day, and it was not just the physical exertion that we wanted to avoid.

What we didn't know was that this day would change our lives forever.

My mother had recently remarried, and we were joining my mom, stepdad, stepsister, Jenna, and her kids for the day. Sara spent most of the day hiking with Jenna while I played with her kids and talked to my parents. Jenna and Sara had developed a great relationship in a short time, and the topic of kids came up on their hike. Jenna asked Sara if we wanted kids without judgment in her voice, but rather out of genuine concern. After all these years, Sara finally felt comfortable sharing our news with family for the first time.

"We've been trying for ten years, and nothing's worked. We're considering adoption, but I want to do a few more rounds of IVF before starting that process." Sara didn't expect Jenna's next response.

"You're family. I'd be happy to be your surrogate," Jenna selflessly offered.

Not knowing Jenna that long, Sara didn't think Jenna was serious or that she fully understood what she was offering. Jenna had her two children when she was young and got pregnant really easily. There was no way she knew the physical and mental toll that fertility treatments entailed. Sara was so sure Jenna wasn't serious that she didn't even mention that part of the conversation to me.

A week later, we received a call from Jenna that changed our lives forever.

"I spoke with my husband, my kids, and my boss and did a ton of research. We're really excited to be your surrogate!"

Jenna was definitely serious. In her words:

"Sara and Ben's fertility struggle became something we were not allowed to talk about with family, but Sara was always easy to talk to. I'm glad she felt the same way about me at that moment, and I'll forever be grateful that she did so on our hike in the Grand Canyon.

After returning home from the Grand Canyon, I talked with my husband, Jared, to see if this was something we both would be willing to do. He said, "Absolutely." We decided that giving a year of our lives to help create a family was a small price for the return. Little did we know that it would be more like three years, but our feelings stayed the same and will forever with the gift that is Hugh," said Jenna.

I didn't know what to say when Sara told me about Jenna's offer because I didn't think it was real. We had gone through six rounds of IVF with one of the best doctors in the world, alongside several other natural procedures, but had never considered surrogacy. We knew about surrogacy and didn't really explore it as an option. We had planned to keep going through our fertility options and try the embryos we had created, and then try adoption. Her offer set our minds racing.

As the oldest of six, I had always felt it was my responsibility to help my family. To take care of them, not the other way around. I told Sara that we couldn't accept Jenna's offer.

"We can't. How could we ever repay Jenna for that…for giving us a life? We can't accept that kind of gift."

I worried about everything that could have possibly gone wrong. Jenna was willing to put her own health at risk so that we could have a child. How could I let that happen? Sara and I decided to consult with our fertility doctor before making any decisions about taking Jenna up on her offer.

California has a specific set of rules and laws around surrogacy, and part of that process is a professional, third-party evaluation of Jenna's health and well-being. I was ok starting there and seeing where it led.

Throughout our infertility treatments, I was painfully aware of how Sara was being affected hormonally. It was brutal. I hated the idea of putting someone we loved through that, followed by the physical toll of pregnancy and then postpartum. Jenna had children of her own, but the process of preparing for surrogacy was completely new to her, and I was concerned.

"Sara and Ben flew me out from Tucson to LA to see if I would even qualify to be a surrogate. Sara kept saying things to the effect that I had no idea what I was getting myself into. I had given birth to two children. I really thought she needed to cut me some slack. However, she was right.

I went through multiple tests (some more painful than others), and the doctor told me I had a beautiful uterus (what a compliment!). Then, the hormone shots came. I had never had to give myself an injection and was a bit nervous. The day of my first injection, I was at my stepmom's house, and she offered to give it to me. However, I knew I had to figure this out because it would be four months of hormone shots.

But there was never a question of whether this was worth it." ~ Jenna

After hearing the doctor's report, it became real. We had to think about what this really meant. I had to come to terms with accepting a gift that I could never repay. I struggled with the decision.

Ultimately, I had to reverse the situation and put myself in Jenna's shoes. Was I willing to do anything to help my family…to see them happy and realize their dreams? That's what I love doing most. I had to get comfortable that this was something Jenna wanted to do; something out of love, not obligation. It was a gift, pure, that I could finally accept.

Our First Surrogacy Attempt – by Sara

It took months to gather all of Jenna's results, medical records, psychological clearance, legal contracts, and hormone medications. Jenna had moved to a small town in northern Arizona without a fertility clinic, so for each weekly doctor visit, she drove herself four hours each way to Phoenix, dedicating more than eight hours of her day to every appointment. Jenna sacrificed more than anyone reading this book could possibly comprehend.

Finally, the doctor confirmed that Jenna was ready for the transfer, and we flew her to Los Angeles for the procedure. For the first time in years, Ben and I felt hope, only to be met with yet another crushing blow.

"The day of the embryo transfer, I was excited. I knew we were going to have a beautiful baby together – all three of us: Ben, Sara, and me. Unfortunately, nothing could prepare me for the blow of finding out about two weeks later that it didn't work.

My world was rocked. Getting pregnant with my children had been so easy for me. My own children are under thirteen months apart, not by accident but because when my husband and I wanted to get pregnant, it just happened. I felt pain, not only for the feelings of disappointment that I knew I had brought on Sara and Ben, but the feeling that came with knowing so many go through the heartache of infertility, nearly consumed me. It took some time for us all to feel ready to try again.

We did eventually try again, but this time my body was not responding to the hormone shots, so the doctor took me off the shots and we waited several cycles. We finally tried again a third time. When the day for the transfer came again, I was hopeful and optimistic.

After the transfer, Sara and Ben took me to a beautiful beach club to get some food and sit by the water. On the way there, I felt motion sickness! I had never been so happy to feel sick...I knew at that moment it worked! The next three months of sickness didn't even bother me. It might have bothered the car behind me when I stuck my head out of the passenger side window to throw up, but I still couldn't believe this was happening, and joy filled my soul." ~ Jenna

The Worst Day of Our Lives – by Sara

Ben and I were incredibly grateful to Jenna and her family in ways that are impossible to express. The emotions that come with surrogacy are complex, complicated, and messy for all parties involved, and there were times when I felt strangely angry and jealous that I wasn't the one pregnant. I was the one who was supposed to be experiencing the morning sickness and cravings. I was supposed to be the one who felt our baby's first little movements. I had envisioned my pregnancy for years and all the life experiences that came with it, and now I was finally an expectant mother; I wasn't experiencing anything that I had expected. I thought I would be the one getting pampered, but instead, I was pampering Jenna (which I absolutely loved doing), but I also resented that it wasn't me. This pregnancy wasn't at all what I had imagined.

These emotions placed Ben and me in a very challenging mental space. We were profoundly grateful and in awe of Jenna's sacrifice, yet we were also grieving the life experience we had always envisioned that having a baby would bring. How could I feel any resentment toward her? How could I be so selfish? Fortunately, I had a great therapist I worked with throughout the process. While I'm not proud of many of the emotions I had during our experience, they were very real.

One of the hardest times of our lives happened 17 weeks into our pregnancy.

I was in my therapist's office, sharing how I was struggling with emotions toward Jenna and our surrogacy experience. My phone started ringing, and when I saw it was Jenna, I declined the call.

"Are you sure you don't want to pick that up?" inquired my therapist.

I rarely took phone calls during my therapy sessions. "Nope."

The ringing started again. I turned my phone over and declined her call again. I'd call her back after my appointment when I was in a better headspace.

Two minutes later, Ben called. It was 2 p.m. on a Wednesday, and Ben rarely called me from work. This time, I picked up, my heart racing. This couldn't be good.

"Jenna's hemorrhaging in the ER. She's not sure if our baby's okay. Come meet me now," Ben's voice was shaking.

My stomach dropped. Jenna was well into her second trimester, and everything had been looking great. She had been extremely cautious during the pregnancy, and our doctors had been monitoring her weekly. How could this be happening?

I felt like I was going to throw up. I had just spent the past hour complaining about how emotionally exhausted I was from taking care of the amazing woman who was carrying our child, and now she was in the ER, hemorrhaging. *What was wrong with me?*

I picked up Ben from work, and we drove home together in silence, not knowing what to do next. Jenna lived a 9-hour drive from our house in Los Angeles. Should we drive there? Book flights? We called Jenna's husband, Jared, and asked what he wanted us to do. The doctor didn't know why Jenna was hemorrhaging or if she or our baby would be okay. Jared recommended we stay in LA until the doctor had more information. We were completely helpless.

Ben and I stared at each other, not knowing what to say, terrified that we may lose our baby. Had we made the right decision even to pursue surrogacy? We were so desperate to be parents and had finally felt hope. Jenna was now 17 weeks along…we had all worked so hard to get this far. We couldn't believe it could possibly slip away.

Jenna continued to bleed the rest of the night and into the next day. She saw different doctors; no one could help. As the bleeding continued through the second day, we started worrying not just about our baby's life but about Jenna's life as well. We were at a complete loss. We were heartbroken, thinking we were losing our baby, but if Jenna lost her life doing this for us, we could never forgive ourselves. She had a husband and two kids; what would they do? Ben and I couldn't sleep or eat, and I blamed myself that she was suffering. It should have been me.

By some miracle, both Jenna and our baby were okay. We were shocked. Ben and I felt numb…we were relieved Jenna was still pregnant, but also felt incredibly guilty that she and her family had suffered so much. We still had 23 weeks left in the pregnancy…what else could go wrong?

While every birth is a miracle, some births take more miracles than one. Surrogacy is full of intense emotions: hope, excitement, fear, gratitude, jealousy (who knew?), and joy, and they're often all mixed together. Even though I wasn't physically carrying our baby, my hormone levels were still all over the place due to our high levels of stress, sleepless nights, and worry.

"We're expecting!" - by Sara

I had just started my second martini when I decided it was a good time to share our news with our close friends and coworkers. "We're expecting!" I announced. Liquid confidence! Everyone's eyes went immediately from my face to my hand holding a martini to my not-pregnant belly. I quickly clarified, "We could never get pregnant, and my amazing sister-in-law is carrying our baby." Our friends slowly began to cheer. Tears were shed, and bubbles were ordered. We finally did it!

I had been terrified to tell anyone we were expecting. There had been so many difficulties getting pregnant, and then with Jenna's ER scare, we didn't want to share the news unless we were absolutely certain it would really happen, knowing full well complications could still occur. We had been so private about our fertility struggle that most people didn't even know we were trying. To now share that we were expecting and that our sister-in-law was our surrogate with our genetic child…what would people think? I didn't have any additional emotional bandwidth to feel judged or answer insensitive questions.

What came as a complete shock was that when we started sharing, amazing things happened…our friends started sharing their stories. Many had health issues they struggled with that we never knew about, including thyroid issues, depression, cancer, ADHD, and diabetes…all linked to hormone disruption. Surprisingly, almost every single person we told had either struggled with infertility or knew someone who had struggled. It was a great reminder of what we had learned earlier; being vulnerable brought us our children, and now, created even deeper relationships with friends and family. We weren't alone.

The BIG Day

May 28 was approaching (Hugh's due date), and we couldn't believe it was finally happening. There were still some logistical challenges around bringing Hugh into the world that we had to figure out. Jenna lived in Arizona, where surrogacy was illegal at the time. If Hugh were to be born in Arizona, we would have to go through a formal adoption process for him to be ours, even though he was our child genetically. We needed him to be born in California, which was a huge ask and sacrifice for Jenna and her family.

Jenna needed to come to LA weeks prior to the due date (and would need to drive, as flying isn't recommended late during pregnancy) and give birth in California. She needed to come to LA in early May, which meant she had to pull her two children out of elementary school early, and they didn't get to finish their school year with their friends. Jenna had already started having minor contractions, and her doctor didn't recommend that she drive herself that far. Jared drove her and their kids eight hours to LA and then flew back to Arizona to return to work. He made that trip several times that month and took his vacation time to be with Jenna for Hugh's birth and her recovery. Jared's support through her three surrogacy attempts, multiple surgeries, her health scare in the ER, and all of the other pregnancy needs is truly remarkable. There aren't words to express how much we appreciate and admire him.

Another thing we didn't consider with surrogacy was our height differences. I'm 5'11", and Ben is even taller. Jenna is 5'7" and petite. Hugh kept growing during the pregnancy, and he was on track to be over 10 pounds. Our doctor was concerned about Jenna's ability to deliver him vaginally, so she scheduled an early C-section. Jenna hadn't had a C-section with her other two children and had no clue what to expect. The date was set. Hugh would be born on May 23rd.

Jenna's husband and kids, as well as Jenna's dad and stepmom (Ben's mom), came to Los Angeles for the big day. We were all excited, although still somewhat apprehensive. Because Jenna needed a C-section, which required an operating room with limited space, we were told only one of us could be in the operating room with her.

We all wanted to be together for Hugh's birth. I wanted to be there to help take care of Jenna, and Ben and I both wanted to be there to experience Hugh's birth as a family. We had planned so long for this day…this was not how it was supposed to happen. Jenna had been picturing this day for over three years, and only selecting one person to be in the delivery room with her was not how she had envisioned it. In Jenna's mind, the reward she would receive for carrying our baby and now going through surgery to bring him into the world was to see both of our faces as Hugh was born, not just one of us, with the other one worried, pacing in the waiting room. I desperately wanted Ben to be in the room to also help support me, knowing that I would be feeling real emotions seeing Jenna undergo surgery.

Incredibly, at the last minute, the hospital agreed to allow us all to be in the room.

Our Hugh was born at 9 a.m. on May 23, 2017. Ben and I rushed over to meet our little man. Ben gently picked him up and brought him over to Jenna, and all three of us were in tears. He was perfect. In that instant, everything we had endured faded away. Hugh was finally here, and he was more than we ever dreamed.

"All babies are miracles, but to be part of a miracle is a gift. Hugh is a gift, and in the time that has passed, Sara and Ben have never taken their gifts for granted. They love their children fiercely and with their whole hearts." —Jenna

---

CHAPTER 3

Giving Grace

"Surrogacy is the greatest gift in the world. It's a selfless act that transforms entire families. My sister-in-law Jenna and my sister Michelle, along with their families, made incredible sacrifices. Beyond the physical toll of pregnancy, there were also complex emotions that we never fully anticipated. I truly can't imagine a greater expression of love." —Sara

The Call That Changed Our Lives - by Sara

We first learned of Michelle's surrogacy offer on April 7, 2018. It was a Saturday evening, and Ben and I were at the grocery store with Hugh, trying to hurry and shop before his bedtime.

"Michelle's FaceTiming me; mind if I pick up?" I asked Ben across the aisle.

My sister rarely called on a Saturday night.

"Is Ben with you?" she asked.

I called Ben over, and we walked to the produce section, where we had better cell coverage. We'll never forget Michelle's next words:

"Let's make a baby!"

"What???" I stammered, not sure we heard her correctly.

"I'd like to try and give Hugh a sibling. I'm going to be your surrogate!" Michelle exclaimed.

My eyes filled with tears as Ben grabbed my hand.

"Michelle, are you guys sure you want to do this?" Ben asked.

During Jenna's pregnancy, I shared with Michelle how much her surrogacy experience had affected not only her but also her entire family.

"Yes," Michelle nodded on the screen. *"Dave and I discussed this at length. Our kids all agreed. We want to try and give Hugh a sibling."*

Tears ran down our faces. We were completely overcome by her offer.

Because we were so private about our infertility, Michelle hadn't been aware of why we didn't have children. She assumed we were focusing on our careers rather than parenthood, and she never asked questions.

When we first told Michelle we were having Hugh via surrogacy (we waited until Jenna was almost into her second trimester before we told anyone in our families), she was initially hurt. Michelle didn't understand why we didn't ask her to be our surrogate. We are less than two years apart in age, and she and I have always had a great relationship. We knew that surrogacy involves so many more people than the surrogate alone; we could never ask anyone to be a surrogate for us.

We had a few additional embryos saved, and while we knew we would absolutely love to have a second child, we didn't know how, when, or if that would ever happen. After everything we had experienced with Jenna, we didn't know if we even had the emotional strength to start the whole process over again. We were so in love with our Hugh and so fortunate to have him that we felt it was selfish to try for another.

We returned home from the store, put Hugh to bed, and Ben and I sat on our back porch rocking chair, processing Michelle's offer. Was this something we should even consider? We held hands, rocking in silence.

On one hand, we were so fortunate that Michelle and her family offered to help us, but we were also hesitant to accept her offer as we intimately knew the emotional toll surrogacy took on everyone involved. Michelle knew we had been considering having a second child and offered to be our surrogate before we even had to make that initial decision.

Could we go through this again, and at what cost to our sanity and relationship with each other? Hugh was almost one; we were absolutely loving parenthood and were at pivotal points in our careers. We didn't know if we had the physical, mental, and emotional capacity to restart the long surrogacy process.

We absolutely wanted to have a sibling for Hugh, but we were also worried about what would happen if we went through everything again and it didn't work.

Michelle's Pregnancy - by Michelle

"Sara is number one, and I'm number two of six children. She and I have always been very, very, very close. We became really close in high school and lived down the hall from each other in college. We got married within nine months of each other. In fact, nine months to the day. Four years later, I started having kids, but Sara didn't. At first, no one thought anything of it.

Sara was super happy for me; she was the best aunt, and all the kids loved her. But in hindsight, I realize now that she had started pulling away. At the time, we just thought she was very busy with her career and had gone back to school, so it was not unusual for her to be a bit distant. We were all so excited for her professionally that none of us thought anything of it. We had no idea that she and Ben even wanted a family, let alone that she was struggling with infertility.

So, as her little sister, when I found out she was pregnant with Jenna via surrogacy, I was sad. My initial reaction was, *"Why didn't you ask me to do this for you?"* I couldn't understand what I had done to make her feel that she couldn't have come to me about this. Ben's mom and stepfather had only been married for a few years at that point, so I had never met Jenna, Ben's stepsister. Naturally, I was very confused as to why she would pick Jenna instead of me. But then she explained that this was not something that she ever felt like she could ask somebody to do; Jenna had graciously offered. For whatever reason, I do think it's easier for people to confide their struggles with somebody who's maybe not close family. It might have been easier for her to share with Jenna that they could not get pregnant.

Of course, once Sara explained everything, and Jenna gave birth to Hugh, we all fell in love with him and were so grateful to Jenna.

I remember exactly where I was when Sara originally told me Jenna was pregnant with their baby. I was driving and so distinctly remember thinking, *"Surrogacy is going to be a part of my life someday!"* A seed was planted in my mind. Somehow, I knew it would be a part of my journey, but I just didn't know how.

I knew Sara and Ben had more girl embryos and had always wanted a large family. The more I thought about it, the more I had to speak to my husband. Yet, I still did not speak to him right away. When I finally brought it up, he first asked, *"Are you serious?"*

I had delivered three children of my own. Our youngest was seven at the time, so we thought we were in the home stretch. Each of my pregnancies had gotten progressively harder, so what I was proposing to him was not something that would be easy or that I was taking lightly.

I don't want to say he wasn't on board at first; he was just a few steps behind me in the decision-making process because I had been thinking about it already for a while. It took him a minute to wrap his brain around the concept.

Then he said, *"We have three choices on this; you could do whatever you want, but without my support, that's not a good choice. We could not do it, and you would probably regret it forever, or we can do it, and it will be a rough year for our family, but then, the long-term of Sara and Ben having a daughter, that is well worth the hard year for our family."*

He was on board. We then talked to our three kids about it. We wanted them to feel like they were part of the decision-making process and shared what it entails. We had what we called the 2.0 talk. We explained that Aunt Sara's body didn't work the way it was supposed to, but my body did. So, how would they feel if we took Aunt Sara and Uncle Ben's baby, but Mom just grew it in her body?

My seven-year-old said, *"Well, Mom, it's bestest to be nicest."*

Then and there, we knew that was what we were going to do. It was a total family affair. My oldest, who was 13 at the time, flew out with me to Los Angeles for the embryo transfer.

I had no idea how sick I was going to be, but I tried really hard never to play the pregnancy card. But in fact, I was so sick every day of that pregnancy. I had been sick for 20 weeks with my youngest, but even on the day I delivered Grace, I was still dry-heaving on the way to the hospital.

Still, I would have so much rather been physically sick than wondering and worrying if I was still pregnant. I took being physically sick as a sign that my body was still doing what it was supposed to be doing. It was emotionally reassuring that the baby was okay.

I was almost 39 years old when I delivered, so my body was just more tired. I was considered a geriatric pregnancy. Despite trying everything to curb the nausea, including acupuncture and acupressure, nothing worked. During the last four weeks of my pregnancy, Grace's birth weight started dropping significantly, so I had to go to the doctor frequently for stress and nonstress tests, which was very stressful in itself. Ultimately, the sickness and stress were a very small price to pay.

Since I live in Oklahoma and Sara and Ben live in California, we agreed that the baby would be born here in Oklahoma as a scheduled induction, so that everyone could be here for Grace's birth. Besides, there was no way I was going to drive to California while nine months pregnant in anticipation of delivering at a hospital close to them. I invited Sara and our entire family to be there for the birth. I became friends with the head nurse at the hospital and worked magic to allow so many people to be in the delivery room. Our parents, sisters, and brother all flew to Oklahoma for Grace's delivery.

"I remember the room being filled with family and love. When it was time for Grace to be born, everyone was there. All of the men were at my head as I pushed, and all of the women were down by my feet. Sara was able to help deliver Grace. I was filled with love and gratitude for my family, for my sister, and for my new little niece.

Surrogacy and giving birth to Grace was an overwhelming, humbling experience. There was so much gratitude and joy. It took a team to get this little one here, and she is so loved. I experienced a double blessing. One as seeing my sister and her husband become parents to Grace, and another by having the opportunity to experience surrogacy, and the beautiful gift it is."

While I love all my nieces and nephews, there's something about seeing Grace that just melts my heart. About a year ago, several of our nieces and nephews were swimming in my pool, and Grace (age 3) and another niece were wearing cute little two-piece bathing suits. I was tickling their bellies, and when I touched Grace's belly button, I suddenly realized, *"That's my connection to her."*

Not everyone reacted to surrogacy positively. I received questions about whether my children would think that I would give them away, too. No, because we've had very in-depth conversations with our children about how this wasn't my baby to begin with, so I was not giving away anything. I was just handing back to Sara and Ben what was already theirs to begin with.

My husband, Dave, who had been a huge support throughout the pregnancy, got a kick out of messing with those people and their crazy comments. Of course, he took surrogacy seriously, and he was well aware of the sacrifice that our family was making for the year. Still, he couldn't resist seeing the shock value on people's faces when he would casually tell someone, *"That's not my baby she's carrying!"* and we couldn't help but laugh.

Ultimately, the underlying gift of surrogacy is love. I felt so privileged, and it was such an honor for me to be a surrogate. I'm so happy that Sara and Ben trusted me to help bring Grace into the world. I don't think intended parents get the credit that they deserve for the amount of trust that they have to put into somebody else who is helping bring their child into this world.

California Made, Oklahoma Grown - by Sara

Our surrogacy experience with Michelle was both similar and different in many ways from that with Jenna. Like Jenna, Michelle and her husband,

Dave, underwent the same rigorous psychological evaluations and medical testing. To even be considered as a surrogate, you have to provide proof of successful pregnancies and deliveries. Michelle had delivered three healthy children. She passed the rest of her tests with flying colors.

We flew Michelle to Los Angeles for the embryo transfer. Oklahoma's surrogacy laws weren't ideal, and it felt safer and simpler to bring her to LA rather than ship our embryo across the country. She brought her daughter, Audrey, with her.

The transfer went well, and 11 days later, Michelle FaceTimed us with the news: we were pregnant! We all burst into tears, laughing, crying, and celebrating together. After everything we'd been through, it felt surreal. Hugh was going to have a sister!

Grace's Birth

When Michelle initially volunteered to be our surrogate, she had three asks. One, she needed to give birth in Oklahoma (she didn't want to disrupt her children's school and also didn't want to drive to Los Angeles 9 months pregnant); two, she didn't want to pump and send us breast milk, and three, she wanted to invite our entire family to be in the delivery room for the birth. As the oldest of six, and then counting Ben, Dave, and our parents, we knew it was going to be a packed room. With Hugh, we were concerned that we couldn't both be in the room, and now this was going to be a party. Ben and I agreed on all accounts.

Michelle is 5'11" like me, and carrying Grace wasn't an issue for her, which meant we didn't need a scheduled C-section. Michelle's pregnancy was healthy despite her nausea every day during her pregnancy. But in the last month, Grace's weight dropped significantly, and the doctor was concerned for Grace's health. The doctor scheduled April 9th, a Tuesday, for her induction.

My entire family flew from California to Oklahoma for Grace's birth. Since everyone was in town, we we planned events all weekend in anticipation of the big day.

April 9, 2019

I stood at the end of a hospital bed and delivered my daughter into the world, one of the most surreal experiences of my life. As I held my baby girl in my arms, I stared in awe at my exhausted sister, who had tears of joy running down her face. She had just given birth to my daughter, and I was completely overwhelmed.

Grace's birth was one of the best days of our lives. Not only did it conclude our 14-year struggle with infertility, but it ended in a delivery room filled with love and joy, with my entire family (14 of us squeezed into the delivery room). Somehow, sharing our inability to get pregnant had brought people together in a way we could have never imagined…our family was now complete.

CHAPTER 4

Hormones, Chemical Exposure, and You

When we were trying to get pregnant, we thought we were facing a personal problem. What we didn't realize was that we were part of something much larger. Infertility rates are rising worldwide. According to the World Health Organization, one in six people, about 17% of adults, struggles with infertility, with numbers even higher in high-income countries. This wasn't just our problem. It's a global one.

Hormone health affects far more than fertility; it's a foundation for how we feel, function, and age.

A growing number of modern lifestyle factors are contributing to widespread hormone disruption, including increased exposure to harmful chemicals, poor sleep, chronic stress, and nutrient-poor diets. These stressors interfere with your body's ability to regulate key hormones like cortisol, insulin, estrogen, testosterone, and thyroid hormones. When these systems are out of sync, it can affect everything from your metabolism and mood to your skin, energy, libido, and immune function.

The effects of hormone imbalance show up in ways we may not always associate with hormones: fatigue, mood swings, weight gain, brain fog, acne, and disrupted sleep. For women, it might be irregular or painful cycles. For men, it may include reduced energy, muscle loss, or changes in libido. These are all signals that our hormones are disrupted.

Hormone-related issues aren't just uncomfortable; they're life-altering. They affect our physical, mental, and sexual well-being, and they ripple out into our relationships, careers, and families. Conditions like infertility, endometriosis, PCOS, thyroid dysfunction, metabolic syndrome, and chronic stress are quietly shaping the health of entire populations.

The economic impact is staggering. Researchers estimate that endocrine-disrupting chemicals (EDCs) cost the U.S. economy more than $340 billion annually in healthcare expenses and lost productivity. And chronic stress, another hormone disruptor, adds an additional $300 billion in workplace losses every year.

One expert working to change this is Jenna Hua, PhD, MPH, RD, founder and CEO of *Million Marker* and one of Hugh & Grace's medical advisors. Dr. Hua is a leading voice in environmental health, helping consumers understand their personal exposure to toxins and how it affects long-term health, behavior, and quality of life.

Dr. Hua's company, *Million Marker*, is a health-tech pioneer that developed the first at-home chemical exposure test, a mail-in urine kit that measures exposure to toxins. Her mission is to empower people with knowledge about the chemicals they're exposed to daily and to make awareness of endocrine-disrupting chemicals more accessible to everyone.

"As a consumer, you have the right to information that will inform your well-being. More importantly, you have the choice about whether you want to exercise that right," says Dr. Hua. "It is up to us to present information as clearly as we can to empower you. We do so while progressively building capabilities to inform action."

Million Marker's work has shown that toxic chemical exposure is connected to 70% of chronic diseases, and diet and exercise alone often can't mitigate the effects. Dr. Hua explains, "Even most doctors aren't equipped to help their patients identify and remedy the effects of toxic exposure. To put it simply, there's a lack of reliable research and education."

She also compares toxic exposure to filling a cup. "You don't always notice the cup getting full until it overflows. If we can control how quickly and how much that cup is filled, we can regain more control over our health."

Disparities in Hormone Health

While hormone disruption affects everyone, some communities are more impacted than others. Research shows that communities of color, particularly Black and Brown populations, are disproportionately exposed to endocrine-disrupting chemicals through environmental sources, beauty products, and limited access to safer alternatives.

Dr. Jessica Shepherd, a board-certified OB/GYN and women's healthcare expert, explains it well: "There is an overwhelming rate of environmental impacts on physical and mental health in disparaged communities. We need to understand that this is an issue that is not getting better. Hormone disruption affects periods, pregnancy, and reproduction and increases preterm delivery."

Dr. Shepherd also highlights some deeply concerning disparities: "Black women are three times more likely to die during childbirth. There are many issues that contribute, but we need to also focus more on nutrition throughout pregnancy. There are higher rates of endometrial cancer, with connections to the use of hair relaxers. Parabens and phthalate levels are elevated in Black children compared to levels in White children. Black communities too often suffer toxic exposure from nearby landfills and the abundance of food deserts in these communities."

The Environmental Health Perspectives also conducted a study in which researchers collected and examined urine samples from 630 children between 4 and 8 years old. They compared their findings to the hair and skin care products their parents/guardians had advised using on them within the past 24 hours. The findings are alarming.

"...the recent use of several different types of skin care products was associated with higher urinary concentrations of several different types of phthalates. Overall, Black children had the highest levels of phthalates in their urine. Other studies have found that many beauty products targeted at communities of color have high levels of these chemicals."

"I think this is a very important study because we need to understand exposures in vulnerable populations such as children," and understanding differences in exposures by racial and ethnic backgrounds can help researchers figure out ways to reduce risks, says Dr. Shruthi Mahalingaiah, an assistant professor of environmental, reproductive and women's health at Harvard T.H. Chan School of Public Health.

Dr. Lynn Goldman, dean of the Milken Institute School of Public Health at George Washington University, weighed in: "Until now, concerns about phthalate exposure have often focused on diet since the chemicals can leach into food from plastic packaging and food handling equipment. But this study provides clear evidence of the links between kids' exposures and a range of personal care products."

The Hermosa Study: Small Changes Matter

The Hermosa Study is a powerful example of how small lifestyle changes can create a significant impact. This study, conducted by UC Berkeley, focused on Latina teens, a group often exposed to more endocrine-disrupting chemicals through personal care products.

For three days, the teens swapped out their regular beauty products, including lotion and makeup, for better alternatives without harmful ingredients like phthalates, parabens, and triclosan. In just three days, their exposure to these harmful chemicals dropped significantly:

- Phthalates: Down by 27%
- Parabens: Reduced by up to 45%
- Triclosan and benzophenone-3: Decreased by 36%

The researchers behind the study also emphasized the importance of education and access to safer products, especially for communities with higher exposure to these harmful chemicals. It's an important reminder that the products you use daily, on, in, and around our bodies, matter.

Hormone Disruption by the Numbers

- 1 in 6 adults experiences infertility
- 70% of chronic disease is linked to toxic exposure
- $640B: Estimated annual cost of EDCs + stress in the U.S.
- 27–45% drop in chemical exposure in just 3 days (Hermosa Study)

In the next chapters, we'll explore how your hormones influence every part of your life, your physical, mental, and sexual health, and share simple, science-backed strategies to support them. Whether you're looking to feel better, think clearer, or simply understand your body more deeply, hormone health is the key.

And the good news is: you have more control than you think.

CHAPTER 5

Hormones and Your Physical Health

After 14 years of searching for answers, we learned our hormones were influencing nearly every aspect of our bodies, and we had more control than we thought. We met with top doctors across specialties, but the breakthrough came when we started looking at our health through the lens of hormone health.

When your hormones are balanced, you feel great. Hormones influence everything from your metabolism, inflammation, sleep, immune function, and even how fast (or slowly) you age. When they are supported, your entire body feels healthy. You have more energy. You think more clearly. Your skin looks healthy, your digestion improves, and your stress response feels manageable. You look and feel better.

This chapter explores how hormones influence every system in your body; what happens when they're working well, how to understand signs of disruption, and how to feel your best at every age. We'll walk through the benefits, the science, and provide simple strategies to support your body's overall health.

Hormones Health Benefits

When your hormones are out of sync, you might not feel like yourself, but you might not know why. Mood swings, mental fatigue, anxiety, or a sense of disconnection can quietly become your new normal. But these aren't signs of aging; they're often symptoms of disrupted hormone health.

Whether you're navigating daily stress, a major transition, or just trying to feel more like *you* again, here are a few benefits you can expect to feel when your hormones are supported:

More Consistent Energy and Mood

When hormones like cortisol, insulin, and thyroid are in sync, your energy is steady. You're less likely to wake up exhausted or crash mid-afternoon. Hormone health also supports more stable moods by calming your nervous system and reducing inflammation, which helps you feel grounded and focused.

Easier Weight Management

Hormones directly influence how your body stores or burns fat. When insulin sensitivity improves, cortisol levels come down, and your metabolism becomes more efficient. It's not about weight loss; it's about helping your body reach a sustainable set point without extreme effort or restriction.

Improved Sleep Quality

Sleep is hormone repair time. When melatonin, progesterone, cortisol, and estrogen are supported, you fall asleep more easily, stay asleep longer, and get the restorative deep sleep your body needs. And the more rested you are, the better your hormone function becomes.

Immune Resilience

Your immune system and hormone system work hand in hand. When hormones like cortisol and thyroid are dysregulated, your immune function can become either suppressed (leaving you more vulnerable to illness) or overactive (increasing the risk for autoimmune disease). Supporting hormone health keeps your defenses strong.

Stronger Muscles and Bones

Testosterone, estrogen, and growth hormone are essential for muscle mass and bone density. As these decline with age, we become more vulnerable to injury, frailty, and slower recovery. Strength training, high-quality nutrition, and hormone-supportive habits help you stay physically strong for longer.

Lower Risk of Chronic Disease

Hormone health is preventive health. By supporting insulin sensitivity, reducing inflammation, and improving metabolic function, you reduce your risk for major chronic diseases--including type 2 diabetes, cardiovascular disease, thyroid dysfunction, and hormone-related cancers.

Why This Matters to Society

Hormone health is often overlooked in everyday healthcare, but its impact is profound. From metabolism and inflammation to energy, mood, and immune strength, your hormones influence nearly every system in your body. What begins as fatigue, bloating, or skin changes can progress to more serious conditions like autoimmune disease, thyroid dysfunction, or chronic inflammation.

These aren't rare issues; they're widespread and growing:

- Up to 80% of women experience hormone-related symptoms during their lifetime, many without ever receiving a diagnosis.
- 1 in 5 women of reproductive age has PCOS, a hormone-related metabolic disorder that often goes undetected.
- An estimated 20 million Americans have some form of thyroid disease--and 60% don't know it.

While the personal toll is significant, the societal costs are staggering. Hormone disruption is linked to a wide range of chronic, life-altering conditions, including:

- Obesity
- Type 2 diabetes
- Cardiovascular disease
- Autoimmune disorders like Hashimoto's and lupus
- Breast and prostate cancers
- PCOS and endometriosis
- Chronic fatigue and migraines
- Metabolic syndrome
- Long COVID and other post-viral syndromes

And what happens inside your body eventually ripples into society.

- In the U.S. alone, hormone-related chronic diseases account for over $500 billion in direct healthcare costs annually.
- Exposure to endocrine-disrupting chemicals (EDCs) adds another $340 billion per year in disease-related expenses, especially in diabetes, obesity, infertility, and neurodevelopmental challenges.
- Missed workdays tied to hormone-related symptoms (including fatigue, menstrual disorders, and migraines) cost employers over $2 billion annually in lost productivity.
- Thyroid dysfunction affects 1 in 8 Americans, yet nearly 60% remain undiagnosed.

Globally, the problem is no smaller:

- The Endocrine Society estimates that more than 10% of global healthcare spending is now tied to conditions linked to hormone disruption.

- The World Health Organization has called hormone-related illness a "silent pandemic," costing trillions in direct care and lost productivity.

Men are also deeply affected. An estimated 30–50% of men with obesity or type 2 diabetes experience low testosterone, which carries emotional and physical consequences ranging from depression and fatigue to infertility and decreased libido.

When hormone health is ignored or misunderstood, the consequences are massive. Families are strained. Workplaces lose productivity. Healthcare systems get overwhelmed. And communities pay the price--in dollars, time, and diminished quality of life.

If we want to improve public health, lower healthcare costs, and empower people to thrive, not just survive, hormone health must become a central part of the conversation.

The Science Behind Your Hormones

Let's take a closer look at the hormones that play an important role in your physical health. These are the chemical messengers that help you feel energized, focused, strong, and well. When they're working in harmony, your body functions optimally. When they're out of sync, you feel it, often in subtle but disruptive ways.

Estrogen

Estrogen influences metabolism, cardiovascular function, bone density, skin elasticity, and even brain health.

- In women, declining estrogen during perimenopause can lead to fatigue, slower metabolism, joint pain, and insulin resistance.

- In men, elevated estrogen, often due to high body fat or exposure to endocrine-disrupting chemicals, can contribute to low energy, reduced muscle mass, and mood changes.
- Estrogen also affects how your body processes fat, cholesterol, and glucose, making it central to your long-term metabolic health.

Progesterone

Progesterone has a calming, grounding effect. It helps regulate your nervous system, supports immune and thyroid function, reduces inflammation, and promotes restful sleep.

- Low progesterone is commonly associated with anxiety, irritability, poor sleep, PMS, and irregular menstrual cycles.
- Progesterone's anti-inflammatory properties also make it protective against chronic conditions tied to stress and immune dysfunction.

Testosterone

Though it's often labeled as the "male hormone," testosterone plays a vital role in everyone. It fuels energy, muscle maintenance, metabolism, motivation, and libido.

- Low testosterone can lead to fatigue, muscle loss, brain fog, and increased body fat in both men and women.
- It also supports bone density, red blood cell production, and immune resilience.
- Stress, aging, and EDC exposure can all suppress healthy testosterone levels.

Cortisol

Cortisol is your body's primary stress hormone, and in short bursts, it's incredibly helpful. But when stress becomes chronic, elevated cortisol levels can wreak havoc on your health.

- Chronically high cortisol is linked to abdominal weight gain, thyroid dysfunction, poor sleep, and weakened immunity.
- It also drives up blood sugar and blood pressure, increasing your risk for type 2 diabetes and cardiovascular disease.
- Learning how to regulate stress is one of the most powerful ways to support your hormone health.

Insulin

Insulin helps move glucose from your bloodstream into your cells to be used for energy. But when your body becomes resistant to insulin, it shifts into fat-storage mode.

- Insulin resistance is a root cause of metabolic dysfunction and is central to conditions like PCOS, type 2 diabetes, and stubborn weight gain.
- It's not just sugar intake. Stress, poor sleep, and hormone-disrupting chemicals can all impair insulin sensitivity.
- Improving insulin function supports not just blood sugar balance, but overall energy, mood, and inflammation levels.

Thyroid Hormones

Your thyroid gland produces hormones that regulate energy, digestion, temperature, mood, and more. These hormones are deeply sensitive to your environment and stress levels.

- Low thyroid hormone (hypothyroidism) can lead to fatigue, weight gain, dry skin, constipation, and depression.
- High thyroid hormone (hyperthyroidism) may cause anxiety, heart palpitations, irritability, and unexplained weight loss.

Because your hormones are constantly changing, it's helpful to understand how they function not just in the moment, but across your entire life.

Hormones Throughout Our Life

Hormones shape your body from the very beginning, guiding organ development before birth and continuing to influence your health, energy, and resilience through every stage of life. When you understand how to work with your hormones, you feel more grounded and capable, so you can make more empowered, informed choices at every stage.

Infancy and Early Childhood

Hormones begin shaping physical development in the womb, influencing brain growth, organ formation, and even metabolism. In the first few months after birth, babies experience natural hormone surges that support growth, bonding, and immune function.

The early years are also especially sensitive. Emerging research shows that exposure to hormone-disrupting chemicals during pregnancy, infancy and childhood can have long-term physical effects, such as increased risk of obesity, early puberty, thyroid dysfunction, and metabolic conditions later in life. Because detoxification systems in infants and young children are still developing, even small exposures can carry outsized consequences.

Supporting hormone health in early childhood helps lay the foundation for physical resilience for years to come.

Puberty

Puberty is the first major hormonal shift most of us notice. Estrogen and testosterone surge, triggering visible physical changes, like breast development, voice deepening, increased muscle mass, and growth spurts.

Puberty sets the stage for bone density, insulin sensitivity, body composition, and even long-term cardiovascular health. The habits we form during this time, nutrition, sleep, exercise, and environmental exposures, can all influence how these hormonal changes play out in your body.

With puberty now beginning earlier than in past generations (especially among girls), partly due to nutrition and increased environmental exposures, it's even more important to understand how to support your body through this transition.

Early to Mid-Adulthood

This is often considered the "hormonal prime," when your body is working hard to maintain energy, muscle, metabolism, and immune function. But it's also a time when hormone-related conditions begin to surface, especially for women.

In women, issues like PCOS, thyroid disorders, and autoimmune diseases often emerge in the 20s and 30s.

In men, testosterone may begin to decline gradually starting in the early 30s, especially under chronic stress or with poor lifestyle habits.

Fertility-related hormones are only part of the picture. During this stage, physical health is deeply influenced by hormone patterns, impacting everything from blood sugar control and body fat distribution to inflammation and fatigue. Supporting hormone health through exercise, nutrient-rich food, sleep, and reducing exposure to EDCs becomes key to sustaining physical vitality.

Perimenopause and Menopause

Perimenopause is the transition leading up to menopause, often starting in your late 30s or early 40s. It's marked by fluctuations in estrogen and progesterone that can affect energy, metabolism, joint health, blood sugar, and sleep. Because perimenopause isn't as widely discussed, these symptoms are often misdiagnosed or brushed off as "stress." But recognizing these signs is the first step toward taking proactive, supportive action.

It's common to notice changes like:

- Slower metabolism and unexpected weight gain
- Increased inflammation and joint pain
- Insulin resistance or blood sugar swings
- Lowered energy and disrupted sleep
- Hot flashes or night sweats

Menopause, which begins after 12 consecutive months without a menstrual period, may also bring increased risk of osteoporosis, cardiovascular issues, and thyroid changes. With the right support, including strength training, nutrient-dense foods, hormone therapy when appropriate, and reducing exposure to environmental toxins, this can be a time of improved energy, clarity, and confidence. Many women during menopause describe feeling more in tune with their bodies and empowered to advocate for their health than ever before.

Andropause (Male Menopause)

Unlike the sudden hormone changes women may experience, men go through a gradual hormonal decline. Starting around age 30, testosterone levels drop about 1% per year. Over time, this can result in:

- Decreased muscle mass and strength
- Lower energy and slower recovery from exercise
- Increased belly fat and blood sugar issues
- Lower motivation and mood shifts

Men have a strong ability to influence their hormone health. Regular strength training, prioritizing sleep, stress management, and reducing EDC exposure can significantly support healthy testosterone production and overall physical resilience well into later decades.

Hormones and Nutrition

One of the most powerful ways to support your hormone health and your physical well-being is through food. What you eat directly affects your hormones and how well they function.

Maya Feller, MS, RD, CDN, a registered dietitian and Institute for Integrative Nutrition faculty member, explains: "Hormone health is linked to your gut and brain health; it sits at the center of your metabolic health and general wellness. Optimizing your hormone health goes beyond weight or diet choices; it's about fueling your body with the right nutrients."

Feller highlights fiber-rich and antioxidant-packed foods as key players in reducing inflammation, which can disrupt hormone function. She notes, "There's a link between what we eat, our environment, and how we perceive our health as well as how we age."

Eating a wide variety of whole, nutrient-dense foods, including leafy greens, colorful vegetables, omega-3 rich fats, high-quality protein, and fermented foods, can help support your body's hormone function at every age. Fiber is especially important, as it supports estrogen detoxification through your gut and promotes blood sugar stability, which is essential for managing insulin and cortisol.

Cruciferous vegetables like broccoli, kale, and cauliflower support liver detoxification and estrogen metabolism. Zinc and magnesium, found in foods like pumpkin seeds, lentils, and dark chocolate, play critical roles in testosterone production, stress management, and sleep quality. Vitamin D, which many people are deficient in, also acts like a hormone in the body and is key for immune and reproductive health.

While there's no single food that "fixes" hormones, a diverse, colorful plate filled with minimally processed ingredients is one of the most powerful tools we have. Over time, these choices add up to meaningful improvements in energy, mood, metabolism, and overall physical health.

Nutrient-Rich Foods that Support Hormone Health:

- Leafy greens (like spinach, arugula, and kale): high in folate, magnesium, and antioxidants
- Cruciferous vegetables (broccoli, cauliflower, Brussels sprouts): help your body clear excess estrogen
- Omega-3 fats (found in wild-caught salmon, flaxseeds, walnuts): reduce inflammation and support brain function
- Berries and citrus: high in antioxidants, vitamin C, and fiber
- High-quality protein (eggs, lentils, grass-fed meat, hemp seeds): needed for hormone synthesis

And perhaps the most important? Fiber. Fiber helps escort excess hormones out of your system via digestion. Without enough fiber, those hormones can recirculate and create imbalance.

Foods to try to avoid:

- Highly processed foods
- Refined sugars
- Excess caffeine and alcohol
- Pesticide-laden produce
- Conventionally raised meat and dairy

With everything, choose progress over perfection. Simply choosing these small swaps can help reduce your body's toxic load, and give your hormones a chance to thrive.

Hormones and Exercise

While food is one piece of your hormone health puzzle, movement is another, and it may matter more than you think. Exercise isn't just about burning calories or building muscle; it's one of the most effective tools we have to support hormone health. And just like your hormones, your movement needs will change throughout your life. What works during one season may not serve you in another, and that's okay.

The key is understanding that physical activity is personal. Your body needs different types of movement at different times. In high-stress seasons, intense workouts might spike your cortisol and leave you depleted. During others, strength training might be exactly what you need to build resilience and energy.

Different types of exercise affect your hormones in different ways:

- Strength training increases testosterone and growth hormone, supporting metabolism, muscle mass, and bone density.
- Walking and low-impact cardio help improve insulin sensitivity and lower cortisol, especially beneficial during perimenopause or burnout.
- Yoga, stretching, and breathwork help regulate cortisol, promote oxytocin release, and calm your nervous system.

What matters most is consistency, not intensity. A 20-minute walk, a bodyweight workout, or a gentle yoga flow can make a measurable difference. Even just moving your body with intention--daily stretching, gardening, dancing, or running after your kids--can help support your hormones.

Exercise should support your energy, not drain it. When you move in ways that feel good for your body and your season of life, it becomes something your body craves and can sustain.

Hormones and Sleep

If you're not sleeping well, your hormones are likely paying the price. Sleep isn't just rest; it's when your body works on hormone repair. While you sleep, your endocrine system performs vital tasks: detoxifying harmful byproducts, recalibrating your hormone levels, repairing your tissues, and restoring metabolic balance.

Even one bad night of sleep can throw your hormones off. Over time, inconsistent or poor-quality sleep can disrupt every system in your body.

Here's how sleep affects key hormones:

- Melatonin, your body's sleep hormone, helps regulate circadian rhythm, but it also plays a supporting role in estrogen, testosterone, growth hormone, and cortisol production.
- Sleep deprivation increases cortisol, which suppresses testosterone, progesterone, and thyroid hormone.
- Poor sleep reduces insulin sensitivity, increasing the risk of type 2 diabetes, weight gain, and chronic inflammation.
- Disrupted sleep can worsen symptoms in your body, including PMS, perimenopause, thyroid dysfunction, and autoimmune disease.

Let's talk numbers:

- One study found that getting just five hours of sleep per night for one week lowered testosterone levels in men by 10–15%.
- Women with irregular sleep patterns were three times more likely to develop metabolic syndrome, a cluster of risk factors for heart disease and diabetes.
- Shift workers, who often have erratic sleep schedules, face significantly higher rates of breast cancer, obesity, and infertility, all linked to disrupted circadian rhythms and hormone dysregulation.

And it's not just about quantity. Quality matters just as much. Deep, uninterrupted sleep is when your body produces the most growth hormone, clears excess cortisol, and supports cellular repair. If you're waking often, going to bed late, or using screens before bed, your hormone function may be compromised, even if you're technically "getting enough" sleep.

Sleep isn't a luxury; it's hormone therapy. If you want to start improving your hormone health, start with your sleep. Here are a few habits to try:

- Go to bed and wake up at the same time every day, even on weekends.
- Keep your bedroom dark, cool, and screen-free.
- Avoid blue light and bright screens 1–2 hours before bed, or wear blue light–blocking glasses.
- Wind down with a calming routine: stretching, journaling, and herbal tea.
- Cut caffeine after noon and skip heavy meals close to bedtime.

Prioritize sleep. Even one more hour of high-quality sleep can make a difference.

Expert Insights

"Hormone health is central to men's vitality, not just fertility. Addressing hormone disruption is one of the best ways to increase energy, mood, and metabolic efficiency as men age."
—Dr. Philip Werthman, MD, FACS, Director of the Center for Male Reproductive Medicine & Vasectomy Reversal in Los Angeles and Hugh & Grace Medical Advisor.

Dr. Werthman highlights what many men experience but don't recognize: gradual hormonal shifts, especially testosterone decline, can impact physical strength, endurance, metabolism, and motivation years before most men realize. These changes are often written off as "normal aging," but they're not inevitable. Through intentional lifestyle changes and personalized care, men can extend their physical vitality and preserve strength well into their later decades.

Hormone health also plays a central role in human optimization and longevity. It's not just about living longer; it's about staying active, resilient, and mentally sharp as you age.

"Hormones are central to how we age. When they're optimized, they support cellular repair, cognitive clarity, energy, and metabolic health, making it possible to not only extend lifespan, but enhance your healthspan."
—Dr. Fady Hannah-Shmouni, MD, FRCPC, Clinical Endocrinologist & Genomic Medicine Specialist

---

Dr. Hannah-Shmouni's work connects hormone optimization with biological resilience, slower cellular aging, better metabolic function, improved brain health, and reduced risk of chronic disease. Supporting your hormone health today can help you feel better now and age more vibrantly in the future.

Simple Swaps

While these everyday actions may seem small, over time, they'll help lower your toxic load, regulate stress, and give your body the tools it needs to feel better.

Swap plastic for glass. Use glass or stainless steel instead of plastic containers, especially when heating food or drinks.

Upgrade to hormone-supportive personal care products with transparent, toxin-free ingredients. Many soaps, shampoos, and lotions contain parabens, phthalates, and synthetic fragrance, ingredients linked to hormone disruption.

- Prioritize whole foods. A nutrient-dense, fiber-rich diet helps regulate blood sugar, reduce inflammation, and support hormone detox through the gut.
- Protect your sleep. A consistent sleep schedule, screen-free wind-down routine, and dark sleep environment all support melatonin, cortisol, and repair hormones overnight.

You'll find a full guide to hormone-supportive simple swaps in Chapter 8. Next up: how hormones impact your mental health--and what you can do today to feel calmer and emotionally secure.

CHAPTER 6

Hormones and Your Mental Health

During our rounds of IVF, Sara was prescribed hormone treatments, but we had no clue how profoundly they would affect our mental health. With each round, her symptoms intensified. Sara, who was usually level-headed, began to unravel. She started screaming, throwing things (something she had never done before), and saying things that were completely out of character. Ben felt helpless, unsure how to support her, or even how to process his own emotions. We were both exhausted, mentally and physically.

We learned that mental health isn't just about mindset or motivation; it's about biology. Hormones don't just regulate your physical systems, but they also shape how you feel, how you think, and how you respond to stress.

This chapter is for anyone who's ever wondered, *"Why don't I feel good, even when everything in my life seems fine?"* Your hormones play a powerful role in your emotional well-being--and the more you understand them, the more you can support your mental health.

Hormone Health Benefits

When your hormones are supported, your brain chemistry, nervous system, and emotional responses all function more smoothly. You feel calmer, clearer, and more emotionally grounded. Supporting hormone health is one of the most overlooked ways to improve mental well-being.

More Stable Mood and Emotional Resilience

Estrogen and progesterone help regulate neurotransmitters like serotonin and GABA--two of *your brain's* key mood stabilizers. When these hormone levels are supported, you're less likely to feel emotionally reactive, irritable, or overwhelmed by daily stress.

Reduced Anxiety and Cortisol Overload

Chronic stress elevates cortisol, which can keep your nervous system in a constant state of fight-or-flight. Hormone-supportive strategies can lower baseline cortisol, helping reduce anxiety and racing thoughts.

Less Brain Fog, More Mental Clarity

Hormones like estrogen and thyroid support your brain function, including memory, focus, and executive functioning. When they're disrupted, brain fog and forgetfulness set in. When supported, you feel more mentally clear, present and confident.

Better Sleep and Emotional Reset

Sleep is when your brain resets. Hormones like melatonin, progesterone, and cortisol regulate your circadian rhythm and your ability to recover emotionally. Deeper, more consistent sleep leads to better coping skills and lower risk of anxiety and depression.

Increased Motivation and Mental Drive

Dopamine, often called the "motivation molecule," is influenced by hormone health, especially thyroid and testosterone. When these are low, it's easy to feel apathetic or stuck. When supported, you're more likely to feel hopeful, powerful, and capable.

Greater Self-Awareness and Compassion

Understanding how hormone fluctuations impact your mood and mental state can shift your mindset from self-judgment to self-compassion. This awareness helps you make empowered choices and feel more in control of your mental health.

Why This Matters to Society

We're facing a global mental health crisis--and hormones are a missing piece of the conversation. These aren't rare issues; they're widespread and growing:

- 1 in 5 adults in the U.S., nearly 58 million people, experience a mental health condition each year.
- Women are twice as likely as men to be diagnosed with anxiety disorders and major depressive disorders.
- Up to 70% of women with thyroid dysfunction report mental health symptoms like depression, brain fog, and emotional sensitivity.
- Postpartum depression affects 1 in 7 mothers, but many never receive formal treatment.
- Perimenopausal mental health symptoms, including irritability, panic attacks, and depression, affect up to 70% of women, yet fewer than 30% recognize the hormonal connection.

Men are also deeply affected, though their symptoms are often missed:

- Testosterone decline in midlife is linked to increased risk of depression, anxiety, and low motivation, but is rarely discussed.
- Male depression is underdiagnosed, often showing up as irritability, fatigue, or withdrawal rather than sadness.

- Suicide rates among men are nearly 4x higher than among women in the U.S., often due to under-treated or undiagnosed mental health conditions.

Children and teens are facing their own growing crisis:

- 1 in 5 adolescents in the U.S. has a diagnosable mental health disorder, and over 40% of high school students report feeling persistently sad or hopeless.
- Teen girls are especially vulnerable, with 3 in 5 reporting poor mental health and 1 in 3 seriously considering suicide.
- Rising exposure to hormone-disrupting chemicals has been linked to increased risk of ADHD and anxiety in children.

The societal cost is staggering:

- Over 200 million workdays are lost annually in the U.S. due to untreated mental health conditions.
- Depression and anxiety disorders cost the global economy over $1 trillion/year in lost productivity.
- By 2030, the total global cost of mental health conditions is projected to exceed $16 trillion.

Yet despite the scale of the problem, hormone health remains a missing piece of the conversation. Many people are treated with medication or therapy alone, without ever exploring the underlying biological shifts driving their mental health symptoms.

By expanding the conversation to include hormones, we unlock more personalized, effective support for women, men, and teens alike. It's not just about symptom management; it's about getting to the root and helping people feel like themselves again.

The Science Behind Your Hormones

Hormones are your body's internal messengers. They travel through your bloodstream, delivering instructions to your brain, gut, thyroid, adrenals, and nearly every other organ system that influences how you feel, think, and function.

When it comes to mental health, hormones affect everything from your ability to focus to how you respond to stress, process emotions, and regulate your mood. Even subtle changes in hormone levels can alter brain chemistry, especially in regions tied to memory, anxiety, and emotional resilience.

Here are some of the key hormones that influence your mental health:

Estrogen

Estrogen does more than regulate the menstrual cycle. It also plays a neuroprotective role, supporting serotonin and dopamine production, enhancing mood, and protecting against anxiety and depression. When estrogen levels drop sharply, such as during perimenopause or postpartum, many women experience increased irritability, sadness, and brain fog.

Progesterone

Often called the "calming hormone," progesterone helps counteract the stimulating effects of cortisol. Healthy progesterone levels promote restful sleep and emotional stability. But when progesterone is too low--as it often is during perimenopause or chronic stress--many people report mood swings, anxiety, and disrupted sleep.

Cortisol

Cortisol is your main stress hormone. In short bursts, it helps you respond to danger. But chronic high cortisol levels--often caused by unresolved stress or poor sleep--can lead to anxiety, irritability, burnout, and even depression. Over time, elevated cortisol also disrupts sleep, appetite, memory, and immune function.

Thyroid Hormones

Your thyroid affects nearly every aspect of your mental health. Low thyroid hormone (hypothyroidism) is often linked to fatigue, low mood, brain fog, and even depression. Hyperthyroidism, on the other hand, can cause nervousness, irritability, and restlessness. Thyroid disorders are often missed in mental health assessments.

Testosterone

Testosterone supports confidence, motivation, and resilience in both men and women. Low testosterone can lead to apathy, low self-esteem, irritability, and depression. In men, gradual testosterone decline in midlife can also increase emotional sensitivity and reduce stress tolerance.

Insulin

Although primarily known for blood sugar regulation, insulin plays a role in brain function and mood stability. Blood sugar spikes and crashes can create feelings of anxiety, agitation, or "hanger." Insulin resistance has also been linked to depression, cognitive decline, and inflammation in the brain.

Serotonin, Dopamine, Oxytocin, and Endorphins

These are often referred to as your "feel-good" brain chemicals, but hormones help regulate their production. Estrogen, cortisol, and thyroid hormones all influence how your brain creates and uses serotonin and dopamine. Oxytocin and endorphins are boosted by physical touch, laughter, movement, and human connection--all of which support your emotional health.

Hormones Throughout Our Lives

Your mental health evolves throughout your life.

From early childhood to older adulthood, your hormone levels fluctuate to support growth, development, reproduction, and repair. These changes are natural, but when they happen rapidly or without support, they can significantly affect how you feel, think, and function. Understanding what's happening can help you respond with more self-compassion and take proactive steps to support your mental well-being.

Childhood and Puberty

In early childhood, your hormones begin to shape brain development, emotional sensitivity, and behavior. During puberty, the surge of estrogen, progesterone, and testosterone rewires the brain, especially in areas tied to emotional regulation, risk-taking, and social bonding. It's no surprise that this season often comes with mood swings, increased sensitivity, and anxiety. For some, early exposure to endocrine-disrupting chemicals may contribute to earlier onset of puberty and rising rates of adolescent depression and anxiety.

Reproductive Years

In your 20s and 30s, hormones like estrogen, progesterone, and testosterone work together to support your mood, focus, memory, and resilience. But even during this relatively stable phase, hormone disruption can affect mental health. For example, premenstrual mood changes (PMS or PMDD) are tied to sensitivity to progesterone or low serotonin. Birth control and fertility treatments can also trigger emotional symptoms, ranging from irritability to full-blown depression.

Pregnancy and Postpartum

Pregnancy brings a steep rise in estrogen and progesterone, hormones that influence everything from sleep to emotional regulation. While some women feel a boost in mood during pregnancy, others experience heightened anxiety or emotional fragility. After childbirth, hormone levels drop dramatically within days, contributing to what many call the "baby blues." 1 in 7 women struggle with postpartum depression, a serious and often underdiagnosed condition that can be helped with medical support.

Perimenopause and Menopause

Perimenopause, the 4–10 year transition before menopause, is often marked by sharp hormonal fluctuations, especially in estrogen and progesterone, leading to irritability, anxiety, depression, panic attacks, and difficulty concentrating. Some women report feeling like they're "losing their mind," when in fact, their hormones are changing more rapidly than at almost any other time of life. Once menopause occurs (defined as 12 months without a period), hormone levels stabilize, but depression, low energy, and sleep disturbances may continue if not addressed with intentional support like nutrition, hormone therapy, and toxin reduction.

Andropause (Male Menopause)

Though more gradual than women's transitions, men also experience significant hormonal shifts starting in their 40s or 50s. Testosterone levels decline slowly over time, which can impact confidence, motivation, focus, and even how men relate to others. Emotional sensitivity may increase, sometimes leading to unexpected irritability, fatigue, or detachment. Andropause is rarely discussed, and many men never connect their mental fatigue, mood changes, or lack of drive to hormone health. As a result, they may feel ashamed or confused. Fortunately, simple daily hormone-supportive habits, including improving sleep, strength training and reducing endocrine disruptors, can make a big difference.

Later Life and Aging

As we age, all major hormone systems begin to slow, including sex hormones (estrogen, progesterone, testosterone), thyroid hormones, insulin, and cortisol. This natural decline can affect memory, focus, emotional regulation, and even the risk of cognitive decline. Low thyroid function is common in older adults and often misdiagnosed as depression or dementia. Meanwhile, blood sugar dysregulation (due to insulin resistance) can create mood swings, agitation, or confusion. The brain becomes more sensitive to inflammation as we age, making it even more important to support hormone health.

Mental Health Challenges Connected to Hormones

Hormones affect how you feel about yourself, your relationships, and your ability to function day-to-day. When your hormones are imbalanced or disrupted, your brain may not receive the right chemical signals it needs to maintain calm, focus, or emotional resilience.

Below are some of the most common mental health challenges tied to hormone fluctuations:

Anxiety

Hormone-driven anxiety can feel like your nervous system is stuck in overdrive. Elevated cortisol levels from chronic stress or poor sleep can keep your body in a constant state of fight-or-flight. Low progesterone or thyroid imbalances can also amplify anxious thoughts, restlessness, and panic-like symptoms.

Depression

Estrogen, progesterone, testosterone, and thyroid hormones all influence your brain's serotonin and dopamine systems--key players in mood regulation. When any of these hormones dip too low, especially after childbirth, during perimenopause, or due to thyroid issues, you may feel persistently sad, tired, or hopeless.

Bipolar Disorder

Hormonal shifts can intensify symptoms of bipolar disorder, particularly in women. Fluctuations in estrogen and progesterone may trigger mood episodes or make them harder to manage--especially during menstrual cycles, postpartum, or perimenopause. While bipolar disorder is a neurological condition, hormones can act as powerful amplifiers or stressors.

Trauma and PTSD

Chronic trauma can reshape how your body regulates cortisol, your main stress hormone. When cortisol is stuck on "high," it becomes harder to stay calm, feel safe, or recover emotionally. Hormonal dysregulation is common in people with PTSD, and restoring hormone balance can support healing, especially when paired with trauma-informed therapy.

ADHD (Attention-Deficit/Hyperactivity Disorder)

Though often seen as a childhood condition, ADHD also affects millions of adults, especially women, who tend to be underdiagnosed. Hormonal changes (like puberty, postpartum, or perimenopause) can intensify ADHD symptoms by impacting dopamine availability, sleep, and emotional regulation. Some women first notice symptoms or receive a diagnosis during perimenopause.

OCD (Obsessive-Compulsive Disorder)

Fluctuating estrogen and progesterone can influence OCD symptom severity. Research suggests symptoms may worsen during the luteal phase of the menstrual cycle or after childbirth, pointing to a strong hormonal component. Increased stress or disrupted sleep can further elevate compulsive behaviors or intrusive thoughts.

Brain Fog

That fuzzy, can't-focus feeling isn't just in your head. Hormone disruption can impair memory, slow down processing speed, and make it harder to concentrate. Low estrogen, low thyroid function, or blood sugar instability (linked to insulin resistance) are common culprits.

Irritability and Mood Swings

Sharp changes in estrogen or progesterone can lead to mood swings, tearfulness, and short tempers, especially in the days before your period or during perimenopause. You may feel emotionally raw or easily overwhelmed, even when nothing major has changed in your life.

Sleep Disturbances

Hormones like cortisol, progesterone, melatonin, and estrogen all influence your ability to fall and stay asleep. When these are out of sync, it can lead to insomnia, night wakings, or early morning anxiety. Poor sleep, in turn, worsens mental health and throws your hormone system further off balance.

Postpartum Depression (PPD)

The hormonal crash after childbirth, combined with sleep deprivation and emotional stress, can lead to PPD, which affects up to 15-20% of new mothers. While many go undiagnosed due to stigma or lack of awareness, PPD can be effectively treated with medical and emotional support.

Perimenopausal Mood Disorders

During perimenopause, estrogen and progesterone levels can swing wildly, even within the same week. These fluctuations have been linked to new or worsening anxiety, depression, and even panic attacks. Many women in their 40s are prescribed antidepressants without being screened for hormonal causes.

It's important to note that hormones aren't always the cause of a mental health condition, but they often play a role in how symptoms show up, how severe they feel, and how your body responds to treatment. Understanding this connection helps reduce stigma, improve care, and empowers you to have more control over your well-being.

Expert Insights

Hormones have long been considered part of reproductive or physical health, but top medical experts now recognize that mental health and hormone health are inseparable. Dr. Kathleen Valenton, MD, OB/GYN, co-owner of Rodeo Drive Women's Health Center and medical advisor for Hugh & Grace, sees this firsthand in her practice:

> *"Hormones play a critical role in regulating our mood and mental clarity. Imbalances can lead to symptoms such as anxiety, depression, and cognitive fog. By addressing hormone health, we can significantly improve our mental wellness."*
> —Dr. Kathleen Valenton, OB/GYN

Research backs this up. A 2021 study published in the *Journal of Affective Disorders* found that hormonal disorders are linked to a nearly 50% higher risk of developing depressive symptoms. Yet, hormone levels are rarely part of routine mental health evaluations. This disconnect has led to countless missed opportunities to address the true root cause of emotional distress.

And it's not just mood that's affected by hormonal shifts. Your focus, motivation, and ability to regulate emotions are also deeply tied to hormone health. Dr. Valenton shares, "Hormone health isn't just about physical wellness; it's closely linked to our emotional state. Fluctuations, whether due to stress, diet or lifestyle, can impact neurotransmitters that regulate mood, contributing to feelings of stress or even depression. Supporting hormone health is a foundational approach to mental health. When hormones are balanced, people often report feeling more stable, energetic and clear-minded, which translates into better overall mental well-being."

Stress hormones like cortisol also play a major role. According to Harvard Medical School, chronic stress can elevate cortisol levels and shrink the prefrontal cortex, the part of your brain responsible for decision-making, emotional regulation, and focus. Elevated cortisol is also linked to a higher risk of both anxiety and depression, compounding the effects of hormonal imbalance.

Science is finally catching up to what many clinicians have long observed. A 2023 review published in *Frontiers in Psychiatry* reinforced the urgent need to integrate hormone assessments into mental health care:

"Emerging evidence suggests that hormonal imbalances--particularly related to estrogen, progesterone, thyroid, and cortisol--are key contributors to mood disorders. Hormone assessment should be part of routine mental health evaluation."
—Frontiers in Psychiatry, 2023

Your hormones don't just affect your body; they shape how you think, how you cope, how you connect, and how you heal. Supporting hormone health isn't just a physical priority; it's a foundation for emotional and mental well-being.

Simple Swaps

Sometimes the smallest changes make the biggest difference, especially when they support both your hormones and your mental health. Here are simple, science-backed swaps to help you feel calmer, clearer, and more in control:

- Strength train a few times a week: Excessive cardio can spike cortisol, while resistance training supports healthy testosterone and endorphin production, key for mental clarity and mood.
- Surround yourself with great people: Connection is biologically regulating. Positive relationships help lower cortisol and increase oxytocin, which supports emotional stability. If possible, create distance from relationships that consistently cause stress or leave you feeling depleted, your nervous system notices.
- Curate your digital diet: Follow content that educates, uplifts, or soothes your nervous system, and mute or unfollow anything that triggers stress, anxiety, or comparison.
- Celebrate small wins throughout your day: If you're feeling overwhelmed or stuck, do one thing that brings a sense of completion, like making your bed, taking a short walk, or tackling a low-effort task. These small acts help boost dopamine and your mindset.
- Do one thing that brings joy daily: Whether it's dancing, listening to music, or laughing with a friend, joy boosts dopamine and supports emotional resilience.

You'll find even more simple swaps in Chapter 8, including easy product upgrades and lifestyle tips to support your hormone health without the overwhelm. Up next: Hormones and Your Sexual Health, you don't want to miss this!

CHAPTER 7

Hormones and Sexual Health

Have you ever lost interest in sex—or suddenly felt disconnected from your partner? Your hormones may be playing a bigger role than you think. Unfortunately, sex is one of the first things to suffer when our hormones are disrupted, but it's also one of the first areas to improve when our hormones are supported.

When we were trying to get pregnant, sex became way less, well, sexy. What was once spontaneous and fun became scheduled and choreographed. Sara would ask, "Are we sure this is the best position? Should we do it every day or space it out?" As years went by, our nights ended with Sara muttering, "Can you tell me when you're done so I can go to sleep?" followed by Ben's loving response, "Are you kidding? Do you know how many other women would kill to be awake for this?" We laughed, but infertility was ruining our sex life.

All of our unsuccessful pregnancy tests came at a huge price, and not just financially. We were constantly stressed and talking about sex constantly, but not in the way anyone would think. Our pillow talk was replaced with strategic discussions about how long Sara should keep her legs up, or trying every position possible to see if that would help. Should it be morning or at night…or both (Ben's suggestion)? Trying to figure out optimal timing took the 'sexy' right out of our sex life.

Benefits of Hormone Health

When your hormones are supported, your sex life can significantly improve. Relationships become easier--physically and emotionally. The benefits go far beyond the bedroom; they enhance intimacy, emotional resilience, and even longevity. Here are a few of the benefits.

More Satisfying Intimacy

Hormones like estrogen, testosterone, and oxytocin play essential roles in arousal, lubrication, orgasm, and physical sensitivity. In women, balanced estrogen helps restore vaginal pH and lubrication, reducing discomfort, infections, and painful intercourse. Progesterone supports emotional calm and better sleep, which both contribute to sexual connection and closeness. Healthy testosterone levels are linked to stronger desire, more frequent orgasms, and higher sexual confidence. One study found that women with optimal testosterone reported not just more desire--but significantly greater overall sexual satisfaction.

Greater Emotional Connection

Hormone health supports mental clarity, emotional regulation, and mood stability--all of which make it easier to connect with your partner. Oxytocin rises during touch, cuddling, and sex, reinforcing feelings of trust. Even small acts of affection can have a powerful effect. Oxytocin levels can rise significantly after just 20 seconds of hugging.

Increased Confidence and Self-Esteem

When hormones like testosterone, thyroid, and estrogen are supported, they contribute to a greater sense of vitality, body confidence, and mental sharpness, all of which influence how you show up in relationships. Women with optimal hormone profiles report significantly higher levels of self-confidence, relationship satisfaction, and emotional well-being.

Improved Longevity (Especially in Men)

The benefits of a healthy sex life extend beyond pleasure; they may actually add years to your life. A well-known longitudinal study found that men who have sex twice a week have a 50% lower mortality rate over a 10-year period compared to those who have sex once a month.

Positive Impact on Children and Family

When parents nurture emotional and physical connections, it positively affects their children. Children who witness physical affection between their parents, like hugging or holding hands, feel more emotionally secure and resilient. One study found that children who received regular affection from parents were significantly happier and more well-adjusted as adults.

Reduced Tension and Conflict

Hormone health improves sleep, reduces stress, and promotes clearer thinking, all of which lower the likelihood of arguments, miscommunication, and emotional reactivity. Chronic cortisol elevation is linked to increased relationship strain, emotional withdrawal, and reduced empathy.

Why This Matters to Society

Sexual health is often treated as a personal issue, but its impact is widespread. When hormone health is overlooked, it affects relationships, families, and even workforce productivity.

- Sexual dysfunction affects over 43% of women and 31% of men, often due to hormone issues that go unrecognized or untreated. *(Journal of the American Medical Association)*

- Low testosterone affects 1 in 4 men over 30, yet most go undiagnosed, leading to fatigue, depression, and relationship strain.
- Just 55% of people report being satisfied with their sex life, even though many root causes, like hormonal imbalance, are addressable. (*National Library of Medicine*)
- A 2021 survey from the American Sexual Health Association found that nearly half of adults report that sexual dissatisfaction negatively affects their mental health.
- Hormone-related sexual dysfunction contributes to increased use of antidepressants, decreased work productivity, and higher divorce rates.
- For women, hormone-driven vaginal atrophy and pain during intercourse, especially during perimenopause and menopause, go unaddressed by most healthcare providers.
- In the workplace, unaddressed hormone health issues (including PMS, fatigue, and low libido) contribute to absenteeism and decreased engagement, costing employers billions annually.

Supporting hormone health improves not just sex but also quality of life, mental health, and emotional well-being. It strengthens families and relationships, and relieves the societal burden of chronic stress, misdiagnosed conditions, and preventable disease.

How Hormones Shape Relationships

Our relationships are shaped by biology as much as behavior, and hormones play a powerful role in shaping how safe, connected, and emotionally available we feel.

One of the most powerful hormones driving connection is oxytocin. It surges during physical intimacy, childbirth, breastfeeding, and even acts of kindness. Oxytocin helps build trust, calm our nervous system, and increase feelings of emotional closeness. Research shows that couples with higher oxytocin levels report greater relationship satisfaction and lower stress.

Oxytocin doesn't just respond to sex; it responds to touch. Research shows that a 10–20 second hug can release enough oxytocin to lower your cortisol levels, improve your mood, and regulate your heart rate. Hugs can create resilience and reinforce emotional safety--both essential for a healthy sex life.

When our hormones are out of balance, especially during times of high stress or low sleep, we can become more withdrawn, emotionally disconnected, or irritable. This isn't just psychological, it's chemical. Your body is prioritizing survival over connection, which is why rebuilding intimacy often starts outside the bedroom.

This is especially important during life transitions like postpartum, perimenopause, or burnout; times when hormonal shifts make intimacy feel more vulnerable or complex. During these times, physical closeness without pressure, holding hands, massages, and back rubs, can help the connection that stress may have dulled.

Sometimes we think we need to do more to feel connected. But often it's about doing less, showing up, being present, and letting your body's natural chemistry do what it was designed to do.

Desire Disrupted

Low libido is one of the most common concerns related to hormone health, and also one of the most misunderstood. We tend to think of desire as a switch that should always be "on," and when it's not, we blame ourselves or our partners. Desire isn't a constant; it changes based on hormone levels, sleep, stress, and how safe you feel.

Hormones That Boost Desire:

- Testosterone – fuels libido
- Dopamine – drives anticipation
- Estrogen – supports sensitivity
- Oxytocin – deepens connection

When these hormones are balanced, desire can feel spontaneous and exciting. But when they're disrupted, due to stress, sleep deprivation, chronic inflammation, or chemical exposure, your libido drops.

When stress levels are high, cortisol floods our body and suppresses the hormones that regulate desire as a protective response. Your body isn't prioritizing pleasure; it's trying to survive. The good news is that desire can come back, often faster than you think, when you start supporting the systems that fuel it. A few simple ideas:

- Getting better sleep (one of the biggest libido boosters).
- Managing stress through walking, therapy, or spending time in nature.
- Reducing exposure to endocrine-disrupting chemicals.
- Using products that support, not suppress, your hormones.
- Creating times to connect without pressure for performance.

Intimacy After Disconnection

One of the hardest parts of improving your sex life can be overcoming the emotional distance that's occurred. Whether it's been a few weeks, months, or a few years, many couples go through times where intimacy is nonexistent. You may have a newborn, infertility, burnout, menopause, health challenges, or just stress. Hormone changes may have also reduced your desire, energy, or confidence and intimacy feels impossible to restart.

Disconnection doesn't mean something is broken; it simply means there's been stress that needs to be acknowledged and repaired. When hormones are out of sync, your body deprioritizes pleasure and connection to focus on survival. But once your body starts to feel supported and safe again, intimacy can return, even faster than you expect.

"Differences in sexual desire is one of the biggest complaints couples have. It's crucial that you not make your partner the problem but that you stand together as a team against the problem. This allows for curiosity about yourself and each other. Think about it as an invitation to get vulnerable and to hold each other's hearts with empathy and care. It doesn't matter who you're in a relationship with; desire problems are inevitable. Working through them together deepens intimacy."
– Alexandra Katehakis, Ph.D., clinical sexologist and Founder of Center for Healthy Sex in Los Angeles.

What Happens When Our Hormones Are Out of Balance

Unfortunately, hormone disruption leads to several health problems that affect us differently. In women, common signs of hormone imbalance include:

- Irregular menstrual cycles
- Mood swings or heightened emotional sensitivity
- Fatigue
- Low sex drive
- Skin issues

- Difficulty sleeping
- Vaginal dryness or irritation

Low estrogen, especially during perimenopause and menopause, can lead to thinning of the vaginal tissue, reduced lubrication, and painful intercourse. Progesterone imbalances can also contribute to mood changes, sleep issues, and anxiety.

In men, signs of imbalance often include:

- Decreased energy and muscle mass
- Fatigue
- Lower libido
- Thinning hair
- Changes in mood or motivation

Hormones throughout our lives

Even before we're born, hormones start shaping us: our bodies, our brains, our identity and eventually, our sex lives. To better understand how hormones shape our sexuality, let's look at how they evolve through key life stages.

Infancy and Early Childhood

Hormones start shaping us long before we hit puberty; long before we're even born. In the womb, hormonal signals guide the formation of major organs, influence brain development, and lay the foundation for the reproductive system. After birth, babies experience a series of natural hormone surges, especially in the first few months. These early fluctuations are critical for healthy development and help set the stage for growth, bonding, metabolism, and future reproductive health.

Emerging research shows that early hormone disruption can have lasting effects. Exposure to EDCs during pregnancy and early childhood has been linked to earlier onset of puberty, lower sperm counts in men, and increased risk of hormone-related conditions like PCOS and endometriosis in women. Because infants and young children have immature detoxification systems, even low levels of exposure during these sensitive windows can matter.

Understanding how early hormone environments influence long-term health helps us better support our children--not just now, but well into their future. As children grow, hormones continue to shape their development.

Puberty

Puberty is the first big hormonal shift most people recognize. Estrogen and testosterone increase dramatically, triggering a cascade of physical, emotional, and cognitive changes that shape how we view ourselves and how we connect with others. These hormones influence everything from breast development and voice changes to mood swings and sexual curiosity. It can be amazing, awkward, exciting, and confusing, all at the same time.

Hormonal changes during this time also affect confidence, body image, and early ideas about intimacy and identity. It's often the first stage where young people become aware of how powerfully hormones can shape their experience of the world and their connection to others.

Fertility

Hormones play a leading role in fertility. For women, hormones guide ovulation and prepare the body for pregnancy. For men, testosterone is key to producing healthy, motile sperm. Environmental factors, lifestyle choices, and the products we use can impact this balance.

One thing we learned is that while women are born with all the eggs they'll ever have, men get a fresh start every 64-72 days when their sperm regenerates. This gives men a unique opportunity to influence their fertility in real-time through better choices in products and lifestyle. Simple changes, like avoiding plastic water bottles, upgrading skincare, and switching to non-toxic household cleaners, can lead to significant improvements.

For women, choices are similar but more nuanced. While egg quality is more difficult to improve, the environment you create for your body is important. From trying to reduce stress to optimizing diet, every positive choice you make supports your hormones and enhances your fertility potential.

Perimenopause and Menopause

Perimenopause is the transitional phase leading up to menopause, and it can start as early as your late 30s or early 40s, sometimes even earlier. This phase can last 4 to 10 years and is marked by hormone fluctuations, especially in estrogen and progesterone. Symptoms may include irregular periods, night sweats, mood swings, vaginal dryness, and sleep issues, but many women don't connect these to hormones at first. Because perimenopause isn't as widely known, it's often misdiagnosed, and it's assumed it's because of stress or "just getting older."

Menopause is officially marked after 12 consecutive months without a period. While some women ease through it, others experience intense changes, including hot flashes, weight gain, and/or reduced libido. Menopause isn't an ending for your health or your sex life. With the right support, many women report greater confidence, better sex, and more fulfilling relationships than ever before.

Supporting your body during this transition looks different for everyone. Some women find relief with hormone therapy (which should be discussed with a trusted provider), while others focus on lifestyle changes--like nutrient-dense food, strength training, mindfulness, and selecting hormone-supportive products.

Andropause (Male Menopause)

Men experience a more gradual hormone change, often referred to as andropause or "male menopause." Many men assume they're just getting older, but often, it's a hormone issue. The great news is that men have significant power to influence testosterone production through better sleep, resistance training, stress management, and reducing their exposure to EDCs.

Expert Insights on Fertility and Hormone Health

Over the years, we've been fortunate to collaborate with some of the brightest minds in fertility, hormones, and sexual health. Two experts we're honored to partner with, Dr. Brian Kaplan and Dr. Mark Surrey, are not only leaders in their fields but also trusted friends and advisors to Hugh & Grace. Their insights have shaped the way we understand and approach hormone health.

Dr. Brian Kaplan, a world-renowned reproductive endocrinologist at Fertility Centers of Illinois and founder of Ova Egg Freezing in Chicago, is as approachable as he is brilliant. His individualized approach to reproductive health is a game-changer, blending cutting-edge science with genuine care for each patient.

Dr. Mark Surrey is a board-certified reproductive and endoscopic surgeon with over three decades of expertise. As the co-founder and medical director of the Southern California Reproductive Center (SCRC) in Beverly Hills, he's constantly pushing the boundaries of research and innovation in reproductive medicine, all while contributing to leading medical journals.

Dr. Brian Kaplan emphasizes the complexity of fertility and hormone health, recommending a holistic and patient-focused approach.

"There's no single answer to this issue. It's a multifactorial problem that requires multifactor treatment. It's a problem when someone proposes there's a single solution. It tends to complicate things."

His practice revolves around the fundamentals of medicine while considering the unique factors that can influence outcomes--like lifestyle, diet, and mindset. Time, particularly for women, is a critical factor, but a well-rounded strategy that incorporates these additional elements can significantly enhance reproductive health.

Dr. Mark Surrey sheds light on one of the most perplexing challenges in reproductive care: unexplained infertility. He sees this in about 20% of his patients, where standard tests fail to pinpoint a single cause.

Sometimes, age or genetics play a role, but often, it's the everyday choices and environmental factors that have a surprising impact. For instance, Dr. Surrey notes that the products men use while trying to conceive can be even more influential than those women use.

"High-performance, hormone-supportive products can help improve sperm quality, enhancing fertility and supporting a healthier fertility journey."

At SCRC, Dr. Surrey and his team educate patients on the importance of lifestyle choices for fertility. They often recommend Hugh & Grace's Fresh Start set as a holistic complement to medical treatments--a curated selection of skin, health, and home care products designed to promote hormone health for men and women. While there's no magic bullet for improving fertility, small, intentional choices in daily routines can make a meaningful impact.

Dr. Kaplan and Dr. Surrey agree: improving fertility and hormone health is about more than just science; it's about how we live, what we prioritize, and the steps we take to support our bodies. Recognizing the signs of hormone imbalance and making thoughtful, informed changes can pave the way for better reproductive health and overall well-being.

Simple Swaps

Here are a few simple, hormone-supportive shifts that can reduce discomfort, increase connection, and help restore intimacy, physically and emotionally. You don't have to do everything at once. Even one change can make a meaningful difference.

- Prioritize sleep: Sleep has a direct impact on hormone levels. Even one week of poor sleep can lower testosterone by up to 15%, while well-rested individuals report 14–20% higher libido.
- Upgrade your lube: Many conventional lubricants contain ingredients like parabens, glycerin, or synthetic fragrance that can irritate sensitive tissue or disrupt vaginal pH. A pH-balanced, hormone-supportive option helps maintain comfort and moisture while protecting delicate tissue.
- Embrace non-sexual touch: Something as simple as a 20-second hug can calm your nervous system, lower cortisol, and increase oxytocin. Holding hands, giving a back rub, or being together with no agenda can do more for your relationship than forced intimacy.
- Create a calming bedroom: Your environment matters. Choose organic cotton sheets if you can, avoid artificial scents, and reduce bedroom clutter to create a sense of calm. Plants like the snake plant, spider plant, or peace lily can naturally improve air quality and make your space feel more restorative.

- Connect without expectations: Set aside screen-free time to talk, laugh, or just be near each other, with no goal or pressure for physical intimacy.
- Rethink timing: Intimacy doesn't have to happen at night. Consider mornings, weekends, or any time that feels more relaxed and less rushed.

You'll find several simple swaps in the next chapter. Whether you're rebuilding intimacy or simply rediscovering what feels good, focusing on your hormone health is a great place to begin.

CHAPTER 8

Simple Swaps

This chapter is all about simplifying hormone health and making it actionable. We'll guide you through simple swaps and routines, sharing practical product and lifestyle tips designed to support your hormone health without overwhelming you. Remember, it's all about progress, not perfection; there's moderation in everything. Don't feel pressured to implement everything at once; start with what feels manageable, and gradually add more as you go. Small, consistent steps can lead to significant improvements over time. Hope you enjoy!

Simple Swaps to Help Improve Your Hormone Health

Shower Routine

- **Dry Brushing to Detox**: Dry brush your skin in gentle, upward strokes before showering to stimulate your lymphatic system, which helps flush out toxins and improve your circulation. This process not only promotes clearer, healthier skin but also aids in reducing water retention and inflammation, both of which can impact your hormone health. By encouraging detoxification and improving blood flow, dry brushing supports your body's natural processes for hormone regulation, enhancing your overall well-being.

- **Shampoo/Conditioner/Body Products**: Less is more. Your shower or bath is a place to cleanse and detox, and your skin is more absorbent to chemicals when it's wet. Hugh & Grace offers several high-performance personal care options that are versatile and help support hormone health.

- **Switch to a Metal Razor Without a Lubricating Strip**: Conventional razors with lubricating strips often contain synthetic chemicals, fragrances, and EDCs that can be absorbed through the skin. A reusable metal razor provides a great, eco-friendly alternative, offering a clean, close shave without unnecessary exposure to harmful substances. This switch not only supports your hormone health but also reduces plastic waste, making it a sustainable and cost-effective choice.

- **Use a Water Filtration System for Your Shower Head**: Installing a shower filter helps reduce your exposure to chlorine and other harmful chemicals commonly found in tap water. These chemicals can be absorbed through your skin, potentially disrupting your hormone health. Filtering your shower water supports a cleaner, healthier environment for your skin and hair.

- **Check your Shower Curtain**: Vinyl shower curtains often release toxic chemicals like PVCs, phthalates, and other endocrine-disrupting chemicals into the air, especially in the warm, humid environment of a bathroom. These chemicals can linger in the air and be absorbed into your body through inhalation. To minimize exposure, opt for alternatives made from better materials like cotton, hemp, polyester, or PEVA (a non-toxic plastic option). These are also durable, easy to clean, and better for the environment.

- **Cold End to Your Shower**: Add a burst of cold water at the end of your shower to improve circulation, increase endorphins, and activate your parasympathetic response, which helps reduce your cortisol and promote calmness.
- **Keep Your Shower Fresh**: A clean shower is important for maintaining a healthy environment. Still, many traditional cleaning products release harsh chemicals that can linger in the air and on surfaces.
- **Ensure Proper Air Circulation**: Proper ventilation is important for maintaining a healthy bathroom environment. Moisture trapped in a closed shower can lead to mold and mildew, which can release airborne toxins and irritants. After showering, leave your shower door or curtain open to allow humidity to escape and surfaces to dry more quickly. This simple habit not only protects your health but also extends the lifespan of your bathroom by preventing damage caused by excess moisture. Leaving your shower fan on for a while can also improve air circulation.

Skincare routine

- **Choose Products You Love that Support Hormonal Health:** When making self-care purchases, prioritize products that support your hormone health and have been third-party tested to ensure safety and performance. Use high-performance oils on your skin to support your skin barrier health. Healthy skin supports your hormone health and can help minimize your skin's absorption of EDCs. Hugh & Grace has several great options for men, women and children.
- **Go Fragrance-Free**: Many products contain synthetic fragrances that often include hidden EDCs, which can interfere with your

hormone health. Opting for fragrance-free or naturally scented products is a simple step toward protecting your hormone health.

- **Choose Versatile Products:** Simplify your routine and reduce your chemical exposure by opting for products that serve multiple purposes. Multitasking products not only limit exposure to harmful chemicals but also save time and money, making healthier living simpler and more cost-effective.
- **Avoid using lavender and tea tree oil:** While often marketed as natural, lavender and tea tree oils have been linked in some studies to hormone-disrupting effects when used in excess. Regular exposure may interfere with your body's natural hormone activity, which is especially concerning for babies and children, whose systems are still developing.
- **Gua Sha**: Using a Gua Sha can support your hormone health by promoting circulation, reducing muscle tension, and encouraging lymphatic drainage, which helps with detoxification. This ancient technique also helps reduce stress, supporting lower cortisol levels and providing a sense of relaxation, all of which contribute to healthy hormones.
- **Choose a Mineral-based Sunscreen**: Many conventional sunscreens contain chemical filters like oxybenzone and octinoxate, which are known EDCs and can harm your health and the environment. Choose mineral-based sunscreens with active ingredients like zinc oxide or titanium dioxide, which provide effective sun protection without harmful chemicals. These better options shield your skin from UV rays while supporting your hormone health and protecting marine ecosystems.
- **Choose a Non-Toxic Deodorant**: Many conventional deodorants and antiperspirants contain aluminum, synthetic fragrances, and other chemicals that may act as EDCs. These substances can be

absorbed through your armpit, which is close to the lymph nodes. Opt for non-toxic deodorants made with natural oil ingredients like zinc oxide, magnesium, or coconut oil to neutralize odor without exposing your body to harmful chemicals.

- **Avoid Perfumes and Body Sprays**: Traditional perfumes and body sprays often contain synthetic fragrances and phthalates, which are known EDCs. These substances can linger on your skin and in the air, increasing your exposure and potentially interfering with your hormone health. Choose fragrance-free products or safer, naturally derived alternatives can help you reduce chemical exposure while still smelling great.

Bathroom Routine

- **Choose Natural Hand Soaps**: Purchase hand soaps made with natural, plant-based ingredients. These soaps are gentler on your skin and provide a healthier alternative to conventional products, supporting both your skin and overall well-being.
- **Choose a Natural Toothpaste**: Use natural toothpaste made with ingredients like baking soda, coconut oil, or essential oils. These options effectively clean your teeth while minimizing exposure to unnecessary chemicals, making them a healthier choice for your oral care routine.
- **Avoid Air Fresheners in Bathrooms**: Many bathroom air fresheners release synthetic fragrances, phthalates, and volatile organic compounds (VOCs) and contribute to poor indoor air quality. Instead, choose safer alternatives like activated charcoal bags, baking soda, or essential oil diffusers to neutralize odors naturally. You can also use a mist of Hugh & Grace's home cleanser for a clean, fresh scent without harmful chemicals.

- **Choose Non-Toxic Toilet Paper**: Opt for toilet paper that is free from harsh chemicals, fragrances, and dyes. Look for options labeled as unbleached, chlorine-free, or processed without chlorine to minimize chemical exposure and support a healthier choice for your household.
- **Choose Non-Toxic Tampons and Feminine Care Products**: Many conventional feminine care products, including tampons, pads, and liners, are made with bleached cotton, synthetic materials, and fragrances that can contain EDCs and other harmful substances. Because these products come into contact with some of the most sensitive and absorbent areas of the body, they can increase the risk of chemical exposure. Choose organic, unbleached, and fragrance-free options made from natural materials to reduce this risk and support your hormone health.

Mindfulness Routine

- **Morning Meditation**: Start your day with a few minutes of meditation to calm your mind and center your thoughts. This practice helps reduce cortisol levels (your body's primary stress hormone), improve focus, and enhance emotional regulation. Whether it's deep breathing, mindfulness, or guided meditation, this quiet time fosters mental clarity and sets a grounded, peaceful tone for the day.
- **Positive Affirmations**: Incorporate positive affirmations into your morning routine to reprogram your mindset and build self-confidence. Repeating uplifting statements helps boost dopamine and serotonin (feel-good neurotransmitters), shift negative thought patterns, and create a sense of empowerment. This simple practice fosters positivity, supports emotional well-being, and aligns your intentions for a successful day.

- **Physical Contact:** Even brief physical contact, like a 10-20 second hug, can promote your hormone health by releasing oxytocin, the "love hormone," and reducing your cortisol. Studies show that hugs lasting at least 10 seconds can lower stress, improve mood, and help stabilize your body's stress response, all contributing to better overall hormone health.
- **Connection:** Spend time with or send a short text or voice note to a friend or loved one to let them know you're thinking of them. This small gesture releases oxytocin, the "bonding hormone," which can boost your mood, reduce stress, and create connections.

Morning Wellness Routine

- **Daily Detox:** Supporting your body's natural detoxification process is crucial for promoting hormone health. Detoxification helps manage accumulated toxins and chemicals that may interfere with hormone production and function. Hugh & Grace's Hydrate + Detox drink mix helps flush out toxins, supports healthy liver function, and replenishes essential electrolytes, helping to keep your energy steady throughout the day.
- **Hydrate with Electrolytes (Before Caffeine):** Rehydrating with electrolytes before having caffeine can help support hydration, stabilize cortisol, and promote adrenal health.
- **Supplements:** Key nutrients like vitamin D, magnesium, omega-3 fatty acids, and B vitamins have been shown to influence hormone production, energy, and mood regulation. Look for options that are high-quality, third-party tested, and formulated without unnecessary fillers.
- **Collagen:** While collagen is great for skin, hair, and nails, it also supports joint, bone, and digestive health. Not all collagen is created equal: many lower-quality options can contain fillers,

artificial ingredients, or even trace heavy metals. Look for a high-quality collagen that's third-party tested, sourced responsibly, and formulated without unnecessary additives.

- **Eat Protein:** Eating a protein-rich breakfast can help stabilize blood sugar, support cortisol levels, and regulate appetite hormones, promoting steady energy throughout the day. Hugh & Grace's Triple Boost Protein + Hormone Support provides 21 grams of high-quality plant protein, 210% of the most bioavailable B12, a complete amino acid profile with all nine essential amino acids (EAAs), and a full spectrum of BCAAs to support hormone health, muscle recovery, and overall wellness.
- **Adaptogens:** Adaptogenic mushrooms help the body adapt to stress, promoting overall well-being and hormone health. These mushrooms may help manage stress, support cognitive function, and boost energy levels.
- **Cacao:** Rich in magnesium, cacao promotes hormone health by helping support cortisol levels and encouraging relaxation. It also contains antioxidants that help protect the body from oxidative stress, supporting a healthy environment for hormone function. Additionally, cacao's mood-boosting properties can promote a sense of well-being, making it a great addition to your daily routine.

Morning Routine

- **Make Your Bed**: Believe it or not, the simple act of making your bed creates a sense of accomplishment that sets the tone for your day. It reduces mental clutter, creates order, and signals to your mind that your day is starting positively. This helps by lowering cortisol and enhancing your mental focus throughout the day.

- **Exercise in the Morning**: Morning exercise helps regulate cortisol, your body's natural stress hormone, by aligning it with your circadian rhythm for optimal energy throughout the day. It also boosts endorphins, dopamine, and serotonin, supporting mood and helping reduce stress.
- **Bounce While Brushing**: While brushing your teeth in the morning, bounce gently on the balls of your feet to stimulate your lymphatic system. This simple habit supports detoxification and promotes your overall well-being. You can do this several times throughout your day for an easy boost.
- **Get Sunlight**: Spend 10-15 minutes in the morning sun to kickstart your serotonin production, which improves your mood and energy. Natural light also helps set your body's internal clock, promoting better sleep later, which also supports your hormone health.
- **Slow Your Mornings**: When possible, incorporate slow, intentional routines like stretching, sipping tea, or taking a few deep breaths to create a sense of calm and avoid morning cortisol spikes. This helps set a balanced, intentional tone for your day.
- **Listen to Uplifting Music**: Begin your day with uplifting music you enjoy. It's an easy mood booster that helps activate your nervous system, lowers your cortisol, and increases dopamine, helping you start your day in a calm, happy state.

Afternoon Routine

- **Go for a Walk**: Incorporating a daily walk can reduce your cortisol, increase serotonin and dopamine, and improve your insulin sensitivity, all of which support hormone function. Walking also promotes better circulation and aids in detoxification, which is essential for your hormone regulation.

Aim for at least 20-30 minutes outdoors to enhance both your mental and physical well-being.

- **Eat Your Meals Around the Same Time:** Eating lunch around the same time each day helps stabilize your blood sugar, maintain steady energy, and support your mental clarity. Consistent meal timing helps support your metabolism.

- **Start Your Meals with Vegetables**: Begin your meals with a serving of fiber-rich vegetables to help stabilize your blood sugar, support your digestion, and promote hormone health. This simple step helps reduce insulin spikes, eliminate excess hormones, and keep you feeling full for longer, supporting your overall hormone health.

- **Choose Whole Foods**: Choose fresh vegetables, fruits, and lean proteins at lunch to fuel your body with essential nutrients that support hormone production, provide steady energy, and keep your mind clear and focused.

- **Chew Slowly**: Chew each bite thoroughly to support your digestion, improve nutrient absorption, and reduce bloating. This simple swap helps stabilize your blood sugar and supports your overall hormone health.

- **Play Focus-Enhancing Music While Working**: Listen to cocktail jazz, Bossa Nova, or mellow music while you work. These music styles can elevate your dopamine levels, enhance your focus, and ease work-related stress, which in turn helps regulate cortisol.

- **Take Regular Movement Breaks**: Move every hour for a few minutes to promote blood flow, maintain energy, and help reduce stress. Regular movement also helps prevent cortisol buildup and improves your mental clarity.

- **Bounce Breaks**: Take a minute throughout the day to bounce on the balls of your feet. This simple movement stimulates your lymphatic system, supports detoxification, and helps promote your hormone health by keeping your body active and enhancing circulation.

- **Add Deep Squats**: Do deep squats for one of your movement breaks. This is an easy, powerful way to support your hormone health, helping to regulate stress hormones, improve insulin sensitivity, and promote the release of beneficial hormones like testosterone and growth hormone.
- **Stay Hydrated:** Keep water on hand throughout the day to support your energy, mental clarity, and hormone function. Proper hydration aids in nutrient transport, detoxification, and temperature regulation, all of which are essential for hormone health. Hugh & Grace's Hydrate + Detox supports optimal hydration while also aiding in the removal of toxins, promoting your overall hormone health.
- **Choose Stainless Steel or Glass Water Bottles**: Plastic water bottles can leach harmful chemicals into your water, especially when exposed to heat during transit. Opting for stainless steel or glass alternatives helps protect your hormone health by eliminating the risk of exposure to EDCs, which are more likely to be released from plastic in warm environments.
- **Avoid Plastic Straws**: Opt for reusable alternatives like stainless steel or glass to reduce exposure to EDCs found in plastics. Small changes like this help minimize your contact with harmful compounds.
- **Eat Mood-Boosting Foods**: Add foods like dark chocolate, bananas, or nuts to your midday snacks to boost serotonin and dopamine, which improve mood and enhance your mental focus and libido.

Evening Routine

- **Take Off Your Shoes**: Removing your shoes when you enter your house minimizes your exposure to harmful substances like lead, pesticides, and EDCs that can stick to shoe soles. These contaminants have been linked to hormone disruption, including thyroid function and overall toxic load. By maintaining a cleaner indoor environment, this simple habit supports better air quality and promotes hormone health.
- **Make Meals a Family Affair:** Involve everyone in cooking and meal preparation to foster bonding, reduce stress, and promote healthy eating habits. Cooking together increases oxytocin, boosting mood and mental well-being.
- **Cook to Upbeat Music**: Play upbeat music like pop, oldies, or Latin hits while preparing dinner. Fun music releases oxytocin, increases joy, and improves social bonding, supporting hormone health. You can find uplifting, fun playlists when searching Hugh & Grace on Spotify.
- **Avoid Plastic Utensils with Hot Foods**: When cooking, avoid using plastic utensils with hot foods, as heat can cause plastics to release EDCs. Choosing wood or metal utensils instead helps reduce exposure to these harmful compounds.
- **Sit down during meals**: Sitting down for meals allows you to eat mindfully, helping reduce stress and lower cortisol levels. This practice supports digestion and nutrient absorption, creating a healthier environment for hormone function.
- **Mindful Breathing**: Regulate your breathing and move your body into rest and digest before meals. For one minute, simply inhale deeply through your nose for a count of 4, hold it at the top for a

count of 4, exhale slowly out your mouth for a count of 4, like blowing out a straw, and pause for a count of 4. Repeat 5 times.

- **Eat with Loved Ones**: Eating meals with loved ones can help boost oxytocin levels, the "feel-good" hormone, while reducing stress and cortisol. Sharing meals with those you care about creates connection, supports digestion, and promotes an environment conducive to healthy hormone function.
- **Incorporate Greens:** Greens help with detoxification, blood sugar stability, and inflammation reduction, creating a supportive environment for hormone function. The fiber also promotes gut health, aiding in efficient hormone metabolism and the elimination of excess hormones.
- **Store Leftovers in Glass:** Choose glass containers instead of plastic when storing leftovers. Glass prevents harmful chemicals from leaching into food, especially when reheating. If reheating food in the microwave, be sure to put in glass or ceramic containers first.
- **Do Dishes**: Doing a simple, repetitive task like washing dishes can support your hormone health by reducing stress and promoting relaxation. Focusing on the sensations during dishwashing has been shown to lower cortisol levels and boost mood, supporting a healthier environment for your hormone function.
- **Take an Evening Walk:** Go for a 10-minute walk after dinner and share what you're grateful for from the day. This simple practice not only helps with digestion but also boosts oxytocin levels, reduces stress, and sets the stage for a restful night's sleep.

Night Routine

- **Strength-Based Workouts**: Strength training, barre, or yoga in the evening promotes muscle growth, reduces stress, and prepares the body for sleep. These exercises help regulate cortisol and enhance mental well-being.

- **Take a Magnesium Bath Soak**: Relax with an Epsom salt bath once or twice a week to boost your magnesium levels, relieve stress, and improve sleep quality. Magnesium is a key mineral for mental clarity, muscle relaxation, and hormone regulation.

- **Reduce Screen Time Before Bed**: Turn off your screens at least an hour before sleep to help melatonin production and improve your sleep quality. This simple shift supports better mental clarity and hormone regulation.

- **Avoid Taking Melatonin Supplements And Opt for Magnesium and L-theanine:** While melatonin supplements can help with occasional sleep issues, regular use may disrupt your body's natural melatonin production. This key hormone regulates sleep-wake cycles. Over time, this can interfere with your circadian rhythm, potentially affecting other hormones like cortisol, estrogen, and testosterone. Hugh & Grace offers a supplement formulated with magnesium and L-theanine, two of the most effective minerals and amino acids. When used daily, these supplements promote relaxation and support the proper function of your muscles, bones, and nervous system.

- **Create a Wind-Down Routine**: Establish a consistent, calming pre-sleep routine such as reading a book, gentle stretching, or light journaling. These activities help shift your body into a relaxed state, reducing cortisol and promoting better melatonin production.

- **Put a Glass of Water by Your Bed**: Keep a glass of water by your bed as part of your nighttime routine. Drinking water right when you wake helps kick-start hydration, supports digestion, and aids in flushing out toxins, all of which are beneficial for supporting your hormones throughout your day.

- **Incorporate Bedtime Meditation**: A short 5-10 minute guided meditation before bed can help clear the mind, reduce anxiety, and promote relaxation. Meditation activates the parasympathetic nervous system, which helps lower cortisol and supports natural melatonin production.
- **Use Blackout Curtains for Sleep**: Darken your bedroom to support your melatonin production and encourage deep, restful sleep.
- **Prioritize Sleep**: Sleep is essential for supporting hormones, including cortisol, insulin, and melatonin. Consistent, quality sleep supports stress regulation, boosts metabolism, and enhances mood. Aim for 7-9 hours of rest each night by maintaining a consistent sleep schedule to allow your body the recovery it needs for optimal hormone health.
- **Choose Organic Cotton Sheets for Your Bed**: Your bedding plays a significant role in your health, as it's where you spend a third of your life. Opt for organic cotton sheets, which are typically free from harmful pesticides and toxic dyes, providing a great sleeping environment. While bamboo sheets are often marketed as an eco-friendly option, the process of manufacturing bamboo fabric typically involves more chemicals, which can leave residues in the final product. Choosing organic cotton ensures a natural, breathable, and hormone-supportive sleep environment, helping you rest easy and wake up refreshed.
- **Invest in a High-Quality, Non-Toxic Mattress**: Your bed is the foundation of restful sleep. Choose a mattress made from organic cotton, natural latex, or wool, and avoid those containing harmful chemicals like flame retardants, VOCs, or synthetic foams. A supportive, non-toxic mattress promotes better sleep quality by

reducing exposure to disruptive substances while providing the comfort and alignment your body needs to fully recharge.

- **Choose a Non-Toxic Bed Frame**: Your bed frame is more than just a piece of furniture; it's a key part of creating a healthy sleep environment. Opt for frames made from solid, sustainably sourced hardwoods like oak or birch, finished with non-toxic, water-based stains or oils. Selecting a non-toxic, high-quality bed frame reduces chemical exposure, supports hormone health, and provides a foundation for restorative sleep.

Daily Routine

- **Avoid Touching Receipts**: Many thermal paper receipts are coated with bisphenol A (BPA) or bisphenol S (BPS), which are known endocrine-disrupting chemicals that can be absorbed through the skin. Minimize handling receipts whenever possible and opt for digital receipts instead.
- **Practice Gratitude Regularly:** Consistent gratitude practices, like journaling or expressing thanks, can positively impact your hormone health by boosting dopamine and serotonin, reducing cortisol, and enhancing neural plasticity. Studies show that gratitude can reshape your brain chemistry and support your mental well-being, creating a lasting foundation for improved emotional health.
- **Keep a Clean, Organized Environment**: An organized space can reduce stress and improve mental clarity. Minimizing clutter helps lower cortisol levels, creating a calm atmosphere that promotes your overall well-being.
- **Find Purpose in Your Work**: Engaging in meaningful work can support hormone health by boosting dopamine and serotonin, which improve mood, focus, and motivation. Positive social

interactions and achieving goals at work help reduce stress and lower cortisol.

- **Make a Positive Impact**: Engaging in meaningful activities that benefit others can significantly support hormone health. Acts of kindness and purpose-driven work increase oxytocin, the "feel-good" hormone, and reduce stress levels, helping lower cortisol. Contributing to a cause or helping others not only enhances your own well-being but also creates a positive ripple effect, fostering hormone health.

- **Remove Toxic People from Your Life**: Letting go of negative or toxic relationships can profoundly impact your hormone health and overall well-being. Chronic stress from difficult interactions triggers the release of cortisol, your body's primary stress hormone, which, over time, can lead to imbalances in other hormones such as insulin, estrogen, and progesterone. High cortisol levels are also linked to disrupted sleep, weight gain, and reduced immune function. By reducing exposure to these stressful interactions, you allow your body to recalibrate and lower cortisol production. This not only supports your hormone health but also creates space for positive, uplifting connections that promote feelings of safety, joy, and emotional stability; key components of overall health. Surrounding yourself with supportive, nurturing relationships fosters an environment where your body and mind can thrive.

- **Spend Time with Positive People**: Surrounding yourself with supportive, positive individuals can boost hormone health by increasing oxytocin, the "feel-good" hormone, and lowering cortisol levels. Positive social interactions promote relaxation, improve mood, and reduce stress, all of which are essential for maintaining hormone health.

Home Care Routine

- **Incorporate Live Plants**: Adding live plants to your space can improve air quality by naturally filtering out toxins, supporting a healthier environment for hormone health. Plants like spider plants and peace lilies reduce exposure to EDCs, while the act of nurturing them can lower stress levels, promote a sense of calm, and contribute to overall well-being and hormone health. Spider plants are particularly beneficial for hormone health because of their exceptional air-purifying qualities. They efficiently remove common indoor pollutants such as carbon monoxide, formaldehyde, and benzene, which are known to contribute to endocrine disruption.
- **Improve Air Quality with HEPA Air Purifiers:** HEPA air purifiers effectively remove indoor pollutants, allergens, dust, and even harmful particles like VOCs, improving the air you breathe. Cleaner air supports respiratory health and reduces exposure to toxins that can interfere with hormone function, creating a healthier and more comfortable home environment.
- **Neutralize Odors Naturally:** Ditch chemical-laden air fresheners and opt for natural deodorizers like activated charcoal bags or baking soda. These options effectively absorb odors without releasing harmful toxins or synthetic fragrances, helping to maintain a clean atmosphere in your home.
- **Be Mindful of Candles:** Many candles contain synthetic fragrances, paraffin wax, and wicks with heavy metals, which can release harmful toxins into your home. Opt for non-toxic alternatives like candles made from 100% beeswax or soy, with natural essential oil scents and cotton or wood wicks, to create a cozy atmosphere without compromising your hormone health.

- **Choose Non-Toxic Home Care**: Traditional home care products often contain harsh chemicals that can linger in the air and on surfaces. Bleach and ammonia are some of the worst offenders, containing toxic chemicals like phthalates (in fragrances) or synthetic solvents that can interfere with hormonal balance. Hugh & Grace's home care line is formulated with coconut-derived cleansing. Switching to non-toxic cleaning products can significantly improve indoor air quality and reduce health risks. Hugh & Grace has a fantastic natural home care line that works and smells amazing.
- **Switch to Non-Toxic Laundry Care**: Many conventional laundry detergents contain synthetic fragrances, harsh chemicals, and EDCs that can linger on your clothes and skin. Look for detergents that are free from synthetic fragrances, dyes, and harsh chemicals like phthalates, parabens, and sulfates. Opt for plant-based, biodegradable options that are great for both your skin and the environment. Additionally, use natural alternatives to bleach, such as hydrogen peroxide, baking soda, lemon juice, and white vinegar, which can effectively whiten and disinfect clothes without the use of toxic chemicals.
- **Avoid Fabric Softeners**: Many conventional fabric softeners contain synthetic fragrances, phthalates, and other chemicals that can linger on clothing and release harmful toxins into the air. These substances not only contribute to indoor air pollution but can also irritate your skin and disrupt your hormone health. Switching to natural alternatives, such as wool dryer balls, is a simple and effective solution. Wool dryer balls soften clothes naturally, reduce drying time, and eliminate the need for chemical-laden products.

- **Limit Exposure to Lavender and Tea Tree Oil**: While often marketed as natural and beneficial, lavender and tea tree oils have been found to contain compounds that can act as EDCs. These oils may interfere with hormone function, especially with prolonged or excessive use. Opt for alternative essential oils or fragrance-free products to minimize exposure and better support your hormone health.
- **Rethink Air Fresheners**: Traditional air fresheners often contain synthetic fragrances and volatile organic compounds (VOCs) that release harmful toxins and endocrine-disrupting chemicals into your home. Opt for non-toxic alternatives, such as essential oil diffusers, to create a fresh and inviting atmosphere without compromising your hormone health.
- **Choose Non-Toxic Dishwashing Products**: Conventional dishwasher detergents and dish soaps often contain harsh chemicals and synthetic fragrances that can leave residues on your dishes and utensils. Choose better options to ensure your dishes are sparkling clean without exposing your family to harmful residues or unnecessary chemicals while they're eating.
- **Choose an Electric Range Over Gas For Cooking**: Gas stoves can release harmful pollutants such as nitrogen dioxide, carbon monoxide, and even benzene, all of which have been linked to disruptions in hormone health and contribute to indoor air pollution. These chemicals can build up in your home, affecting both the air quality and your overall well-being. Switching to an electric range eliminates these emissions, offering a cleaner cooking experience while reducing your exposure to EDCs. If you prefer to use a gas range, it's important to turn on the overhead fan while cooking to help diffuse the gas and improve air circulation.

- **Invest in Water Filtration:** Tap water can contain contaminants like chlorine and heavy metals that may affect your hormone health over time. Using a high-quality water filtration system helps reduce exposure to these harmful substances, providing better, safer water for drinking, cooking, and bathing.
- **Choose non-toxic Cookware:** Choose non-toxic cookware options like cast iron, stainless steel, or glass, as these materials are less likely to leach harmful chemicals into food. Avoid nonstick coatings that contain perfluorochemicals (PFAS) or polytetrafluoroethylene (PTFE), which are linked to hormone disruption, liver issues, and thyroid imbalances. Cast iron can even increase iron intake, which is beneficial for many. For stainless steel, look for food-grade options to minimize nickel and chromium exposure and ensure proper maintenance to prevent metal leaching.
- **Choose Wooden Cutting Boards:** Wooden cutting boards, especially those made from hardwoods like maple or walnut, are often a safer choice than plastic or glass. Wood has natural antimicrobial properties that can trap and neutralize bacteria, while plastic boards can develop grooves that harbor germs, and glass boards can damage your knives.
- **Upgrade to Non-Toxic Food Storage:** Plastic containers often contain chemicals like BPA, BPS, and phthalates, which can leach into food and disrupt hormone health, especially when heated. Replace them with glass or stainless steel containers, which are durable, non-reactive, and better for your health. Switching to non-toxic, reusable alternatives protects your health and supports a more sustainable, plastic-free lifestyle.
- **Switch to Beeswax Wraps:** Traditional plastic wrap is often made from petroleum-based materials and can contain chemicals like

PVC or BPA, which may leach into your food and disrupt hormone health. Beeswax wraps offer a sustainable, non-toxic alternative that's just as versatile. Made from organic cotton infused with beeswax, jojoba oil, and tree resin, these wraps are naturally antibacterial and reusable. They mold easily around bowls, sandwiches, and other food items, creating an airtight seal that helps keep food fresh without contributing to plastic waste. Plus, they're biodegradable, making them an eco-friendly solution that aligns with a sustainable lifestyle.

- **Natural Pest Repellents**: Many conventional pest sprays contain harsh chemicals and toxins that can linger in your home, potentially impacting your health and hormone balance. Swap these for essential oil-based solutions, which effectively repel insects without harmful residues. Ingredients like citronella and peppermint not only keep pests away but also add a pleasant, natural aroma to your space. These better alternatives protect your home while maintaining a healthy environment for you and your family.

CHAPTER 9

Moving Forward

We hope this book brought clarity, simplicity, and maybe even a sense of peace into your life.

Stories have the power to change lives. While this book began with our story, what matters most is how it impacts your story. We shared our journey, our highs, lows, and life lessons, with the hope that you wouldn't have to go through the same pain we did.

Countless sleepless nights, debilitating stress, and confusing health issues nearly broke us and our marriage. For years, we didn't know why our bodies didn't work, only later learning that hormone disruption was affecting everything. Understanding that, and finally feeling like we had some control, was life-changing.

Whether this book inspired you to make a simple swap or make a more significant lifestyle change, we hope you feel more empowered and confident in making decisions that support your health. You have more control over your physical, mental, and sexual health than you may have realized, it's the combination of small, consistent decisions that make the biggest difference.

If you're interested in learning more or would like to collaborate, we'd love to connect. Visit hughandgrace.com or email parter@hughandgrace.com. We love working with great people, brands, medical professionals and institutions.

We are so fortunate to have our kiddos and absolutely love raising and learning from them. As Co-CEOs and parents, they see us working together every day, solving problems, celebrating wins, and trying over and over again when things don't go as planned. Hugh, age seven, reminds us, "There are lots of ways to solve a problem." Grace, at age five, recently told us, "Failure means you can try again." They're wise beyond their years (as my dad would say).

These concepts also apply to hormone health. It's not about doing "everything right," it's about learning and trying a different approach in case what you're currently doing isn't working. Sometimes knowing just where to start is the first step.

From our family to yours, here's to a simpler, healthier, and happier life. Wishing you all the best.

Sara and Ben

About the Authors

Sara and Ben Jensen are the co-founders of Hugh & Grace, a science-backed wellness platform championing preventative wellness and offering products that promote hormone health, reduce chemical exposure, and simplify healthy living. During their 14-year struggle with unexplained infertility, they learned about the important impact of chemical exposure on hormone function–fueling their mission to educate, empower, and offer high-performance solutions that support healthier lives.

Named after their miracle children, Hugh and Grace, the company is a wellness platform offering products, education, and community. Hugh & Grace has been featured in *The Wall Street Journal*, *Forbes*, *International Business Times*, and more. The company was named to the Inc. 5000 list of fastest-growing companies and recognized as the Fastest Growing Impact Company by *Real Leaders*.

Sara and Ben's favorite roles are being parents to Hugh and Grace, the joys of their lives.

Photos

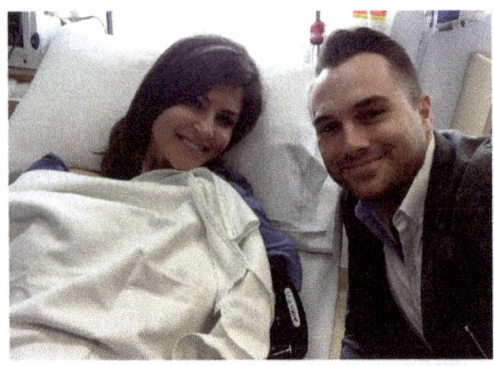

Our first round of IVF

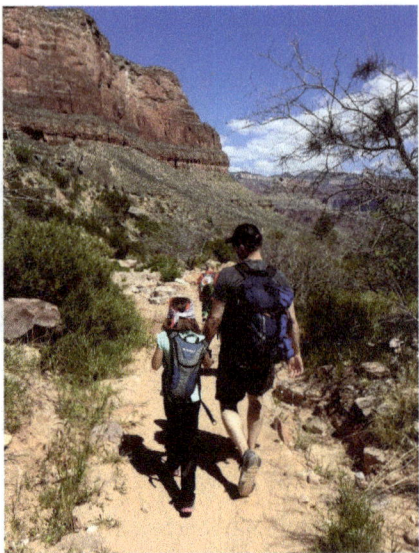

Hiking the Grand Canyon - the day Jenna volunteered to be our surrogate

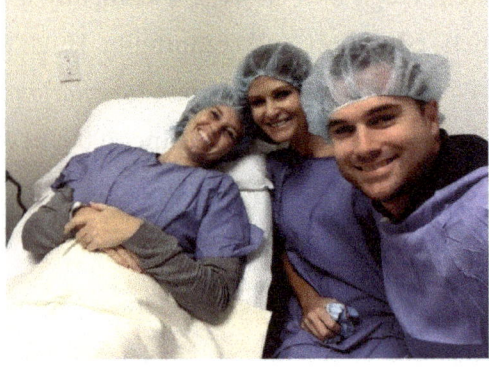

Jenna's first embryo transfer in Los Angeles

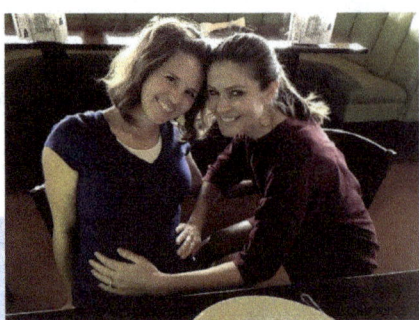

Visiting Jenna in Arizona for her 20-week doctor's appointment

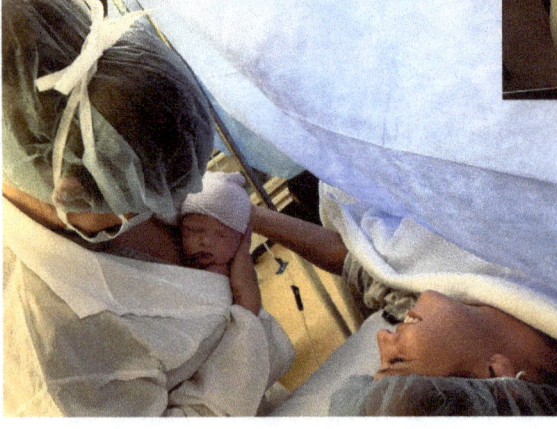

Meeting Hugh!

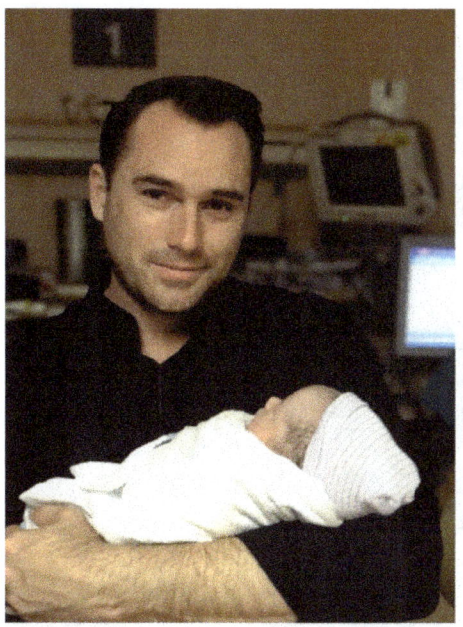
One of the best days of our lives

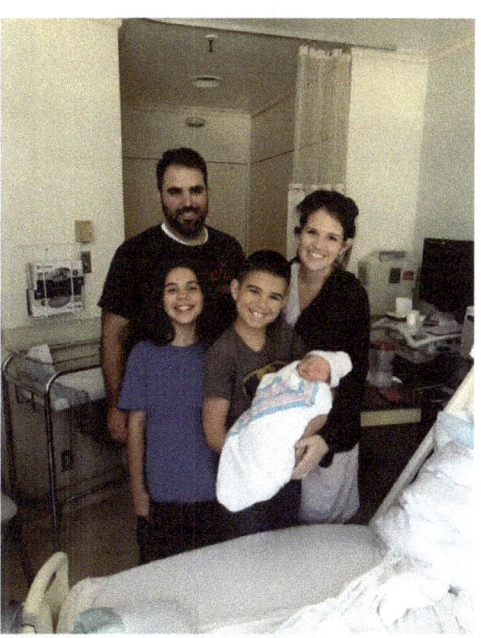
Jenna's incredible family

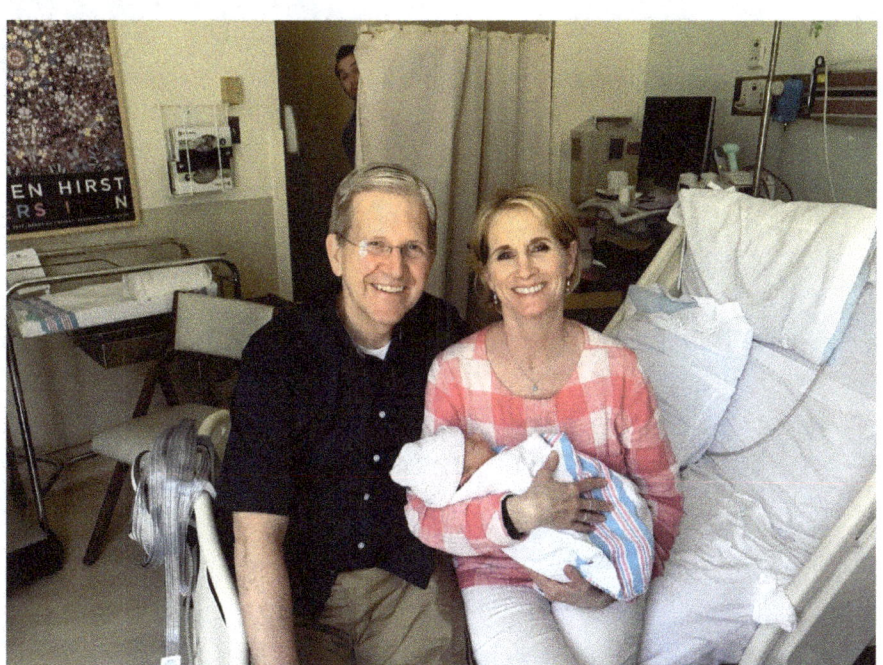
Hugh's grandparents (Ben's mom and Jenna's dad)

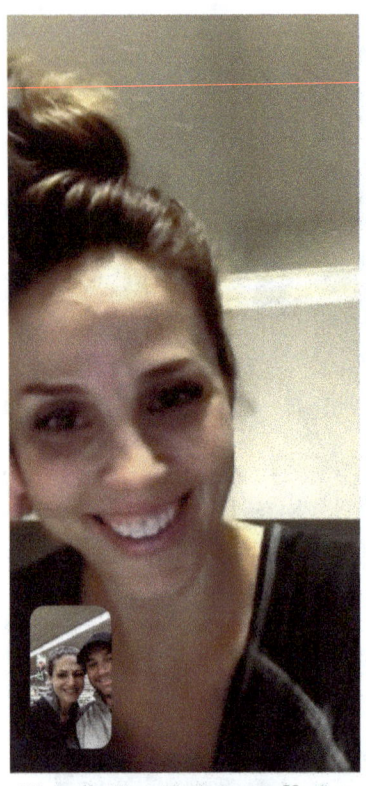

Michelle FaceTiming us offering to be our surrogate

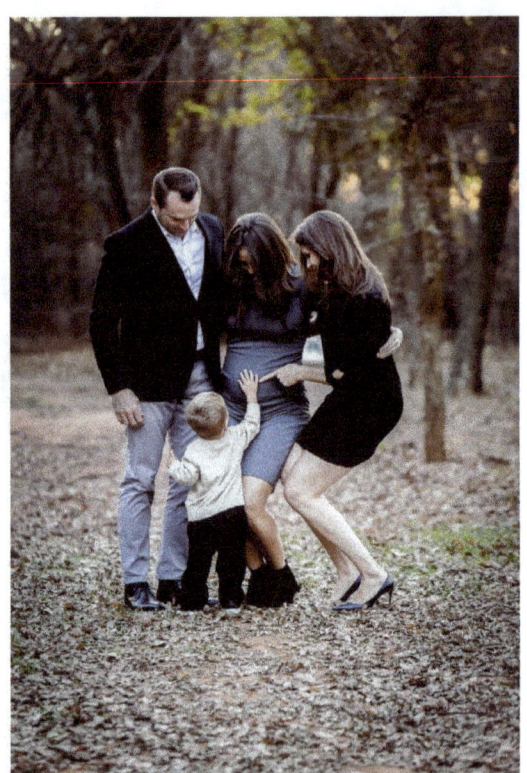

In Oklahoma for Michelle's 20-week doctor's appointment

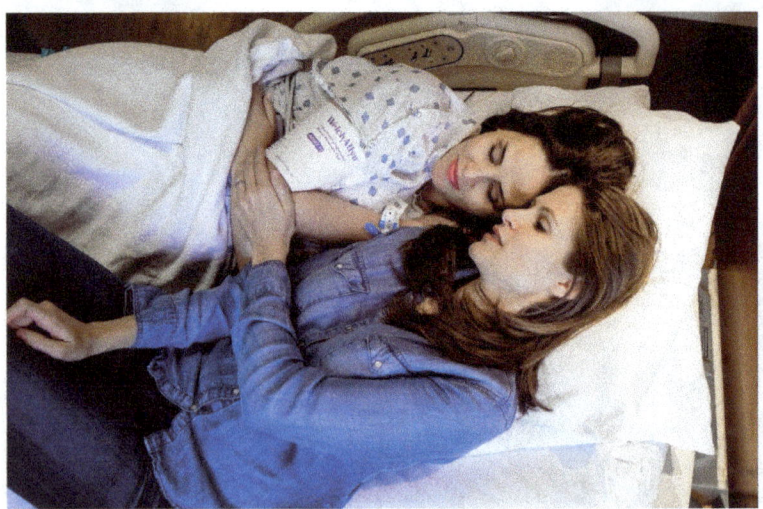

Waiting for Grace to arrive

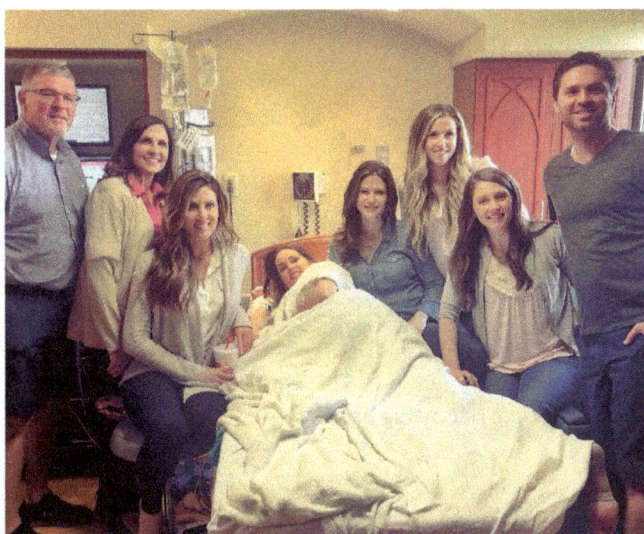

Sara's family in Oklahoma for Grace's birth

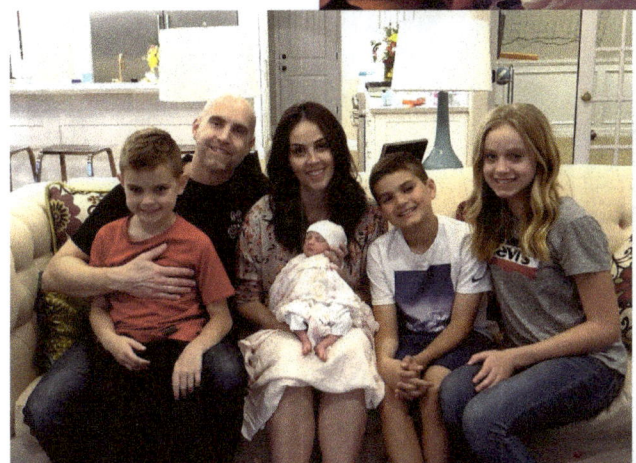

Michelle's amazing family

Loving our Grace

Hormone Health Simplified | 121

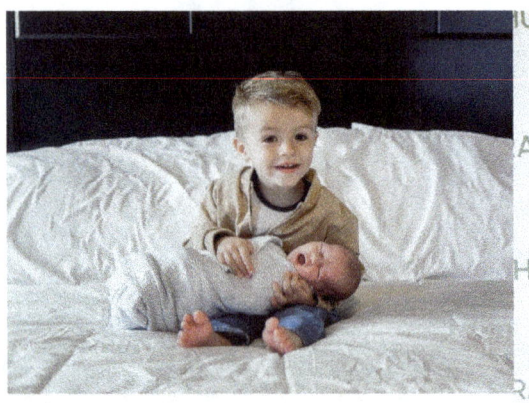
Happy big brother!

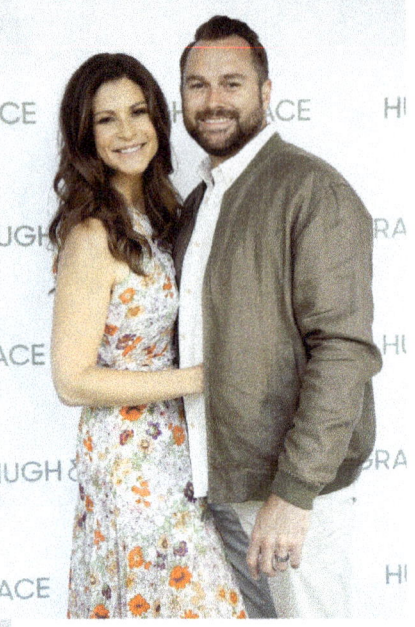
Launching Hugh & Grace!

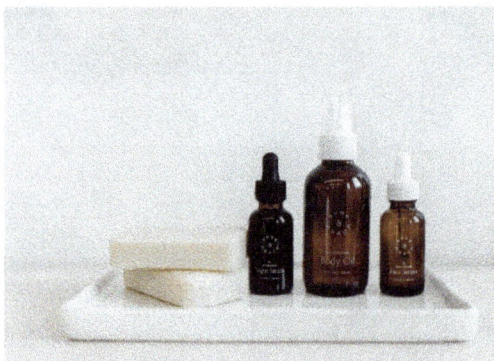
Hugh & Grace skin care

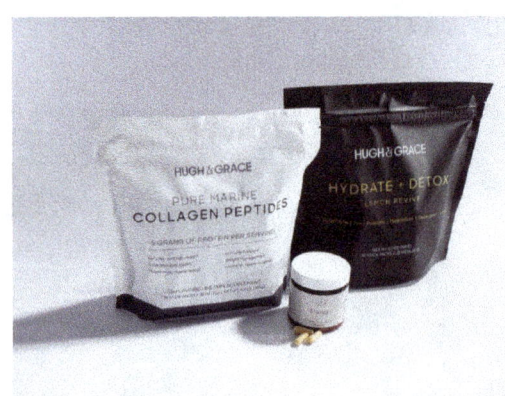
Hugh & Grace wellness

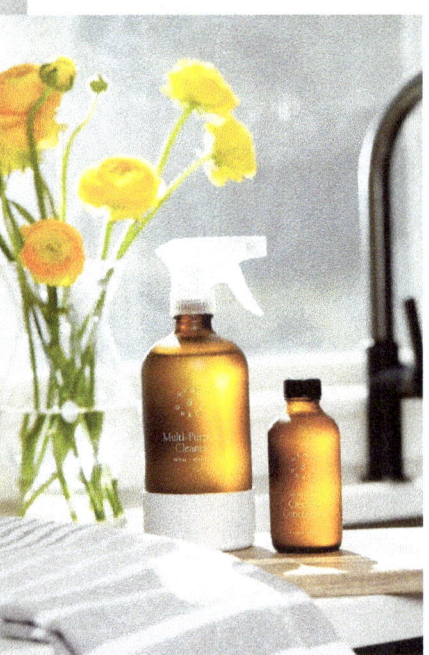
Hugh & Grace home care

References

ACOG. (n.d.). *Postpartum depression.* https://www.acog.org/womens-health/faqs/postpartum-depression

Alloway, T. (2022, January 19). *What 20 seconds of hugging can do for you.* Psychology Today. https://www.psychologytoday.com/us/blog/keep-it-in-mind/202201/what-20-seconds-hugging-can-do-you

American Thyroid Association. *Thyroid facts.* https://www.thyroid.org/media-main/press-room/

Attina, T. M., Hauser, R., Sathyanarayana, S., Hunt, P. A., Bourguignon, J. P., Myers, J. P., ... & Trasande, L. (2016). Exposure to endocrine-disrupting chemicals in the USA: a population-based disease burden and cost analysis. *The lancet Diabetes & endocrinology, 4*(12), 996-1003. https://doi.org/10.1016/S2213-8587(16)30275-3

Bathla, M., Singh, M., & Relan, P. (2016). Prevalence of anxiety and depressive symptoms among patients with hypothyroidism. *Indian Journal of Endocrinology and Metabolism, 20*(4), 468-474. https://doi.org/10.4103/2230-8210.183476

Bloom, M. S., Clark, J. M., Pearce, J. L., Ferguson, P. L., Newman, R. B., Roberts, J. R., ... & ECHO-FGS study group. (2024). Impact of skin care products on phthalates and phthalate replacements in children: the ECHO-FGS. *Environmental health perspectives, 132*(9), 097001. https://doi.org/10.1289/EHP139

CDC.(2024). *Fast facts: Health and economic costs of chronic conditions.* https://www.cdc.gov/chronic-disease/data-research/facts-stats/index.html

CDC Newsroom. (2023). *US teen girls experiencing increased sadness and violence.* https://www.cdc.gov/media/releases/2023/p0213-yrbs.html

Cleveland Clinic. (n.d.). *Vaginal atrophy.* https://my.clevelandclinic.org/health/diseases/15500-vaginal-atrophy

Colombo, G. E., Makieva, S., Somigliana, E., Schoretsanitis, G., Leeners, B., Polli, C., ... & Vigano', P. (2025). The association between endometriosis and migraine: a systematic review and meta-analysis of observational studies. *The Journal of Headache and Pain, 26*(1), 82. https://thejournalofheadacheandpain.biomedcentral.com/articles/10.1186/s10194-025-02020-4

Cox, J. (2025, February 28). *Hormonal issues could cost US economy $200 billion annually.* Forbes. https://www.forbes.com/sites/josiecox/2025/02/28/hormonal-issues-could-cost-us-economy-almost-200-billion-annually/

Crafa, A., Calogero, A. E., Cannarella, R., Mongioi', L. M., Condorelli, R. A., Greco, E. A., ... & La Vignera, S. (2021). The burden of hormonal disorders: a worldwide overview with a particular look in Italy. *Frontiers in Endocrinology, 12*, 694325. https://doi.org/10.3389/fendo.2021.694325

Deswal, R., Narwal, V., Dang, A., & Pundir, C. S. (2020). The prevalence of polycystic ovary syndrome: a brief systematic review. *Journal of human reproductive sciences, 13*(4), 261-271. PMID: 33627974

Eckstein, M., Stößel, G., Gerchen, M. F., Bilek, E., Kirsch, P., & Ditzen, B. (2023). Neural responses to instructed positive couple interaction: an fMRI study on compliment sharing. *Social Cognitive and Affective Neuroscience, 18*(1), nsad005. https://doi.org/10.1093/scan/nsad005

Endocrine Society. (n.d.). *News and advocacy.* https://www.endocrine.org/news-and-advocacy/news-room/2017/10/18/edc-exposure-costs-billions

Endocrine Society. (2022). *Hypogonadism in men.* https://www.endocrine.org/patient-engagement/endocrine-library/hypogonadism

Fernandez, R. C., Moore, V. M., Marino, J. L., Whitrow, M. J., & Davies, M. J. (2020). Night shift among women: is it associated with difficulty conceiving a first birth?. *Frontiers in Public Health, 8,* 595943. https://doi.org/10.3389/fpubh.2020.595943

Furst, J. (2023, April 26). *Mayo Clinic study puts price tag on cost of menopause symptoms for women in the workplace.* Mayo Clinic. https://newsnetwork.mayoclinic.org/discussion/mayo-clinic-study-puts-price-tag-on-cost-of-menopause-symptoms-for-women-in-the-workplace/

Glenza, J. (2024, May 29). US girls got their first periods increasingly earlier over the last 50 years, study shows. *The Guardian.* https://www.theguardian.com/us-news/article/2024/may/29/us-girls-first-periods-earlier

Godoy, M. (2024, September 9). *Hair and skin care products expose kids to hormone disrupting chemicals, study finds.* NPR. https://www.npr.org/sections/shots-health-news/2024/09/09/nx-s1-5099419/hair-and-skin-care-products-expose-kids-to-hormone-disrupting-chemicals-study-finds

Hall, K. (2021). *How does lack of sleep affect your sex life?* Good Rx. https://www.goodrx.com/conditions/low-libido/how-lack-of-sleep-impacts-sex-life-libido-fertility

Hall, S. A., Shackelton, R., Rosen, R. C., & Araujo, A. B. (2010). Sexual activity, erectile dysfunction, and incident cardiovascular events. *The American journal of cardiology, 105*(2), 192-197. https://doi.org/10.1016/j.amjcard.2009.08.671

Harman, S. M., Metter, E. J., Tobin, J. D., Pearson, J., & Blackman, M. R. (2001). Longitudinal effects of aging on serum total and free testosterone levels in healthy men. *The Journal of Clinical Endocrinology & Metabolism, 86*(2), 724-731. https://doi.org/10.1210/jcem.86.2.7219

Harvard Health. (2024). *Understanding the Stress Response.* https://www.health.harvard.edu/staying-healthy/understanding-the-stress-response

Kantoko. (2025). *ADHD in midlife women: Perimenopause, menopause, and hormone shifts.* https://www.kantoko.com.au/articles/adhd-perimenopause-menopause#:~:text=The%20Science:%20Hormones%2C%20Neurotransmitters%2C,regulate%20mood%20and%20emotional%20responses

Kundakovic, M., & Rocks, D. (2022). Sex hormone fluctuation and increased female risk for depression and anxiety disorders: From clinical evidence to molecular mechanisms. *Frontiers in neuroendocrinology, 66*, 101010. https://www.google.com/url?q=https://pmc.ncbi.nlm.nih.gov/articles/PMC9715398/&sa=D&source=docs&ust=1755268818890923&usg=AOvVaw2NyW0bQs8s9GM3Vpjml0FG

Laumann, E. O., Paik, A., & Rosen, R. C. (1999). Sexual dysfunction in the United States: prevalence and predictors. *Jama, 281*(6), 537-544. https://jamanetwork.com/journals/jama/fullarticle/188762

Lee, J. E., Jung, H. W., Lee, Y. J., & Lee, Y. A. (2019). Early-life exposure to endocrine-disrupting chemicals and pubertal development in girls. *Annals of pediatric endocrinology & metabolism, 24*(2), 78-91. https://doi.org/10.6065/apem.2019.24.2.78

Leproult, R., & Van Cauter, E. (2011). Effect of 1 week of sleep restriction on testosterone levels in young healthy men. *Jama, 305*(21), 2173-2174. https://doi.org/10.1001/jama.2011.710

Mayberry, J. (n.d.). *Four surprising benefits of parental love that set children up for a flourishing life*. Georgia Center for Opportunity. https://foropportunity.org/parental-love-and-child-social-mobility/

Million Marker. *Why Toxic Chemicals Matter*. https://www.millionmarker.com

Mulligan, E. M., Hajcak, G., Klawohn, J., Nelson, B., & Meyer, A. (2019). Effects of menstrual cycle phase on associations between the error-related negativity and checking symptoms in women. *Psychoneuroendocrinology, 103*, 233-240. https://doi.org/10.1016/j.psyneuen.2019.01.027

NAMI. (n.d.). *Mental health by the numbers*. https://www.nami.org/about-mental-illness/mental-health-by-the-numbers/

NIH. (Reviewed May 4, 2022). *What lifestyle and environmental factors may be involved in infertility in females and males?* Eunice Shriver National Institute of Child Health and Human Development. https://www.nichd.nih.gov/health/topics/infertility/conditioninfo/causes/lifestyle

National Institute of Health. (2019). *Study links irregular sleep patterns to metabolic disorders.* https://www.nih.gov/news-events/news-releases/study-links-irregular-sleep-patterns-metabolic-disorders

National Institute of Health. (n.d.). *Major depression.* https://www.nimh.nih.gov/health/statistics/major-depression

National Institute of Health. (n.d.). *Suicide.* https://www.nimh.nih.gov/health/statistics/suicide

Papadimitriou, A., & Papadimitriou, D. T. (2021). Endocrine-disrupting chemicals and early puberty in girls. *Children, 8*(6), 492. https://doi.org/10.3390/children8060492

Parish, S. J., Simon, J. A., Davis, S. R., Giraldi, A., Goldstein, I., Goldstein, S. W., ... & Vignozzi, L. (2021). International Society for the Study of Women's Sexual Health clinical practice guideline for the use of systemic testosterone for hypoactive sexual desire disorder in women. *The journal of sexual medicine, 18*(5), 849-867. https://doi.org/10.1016/j.jsxm.2020.10.009

Reiter, S. (2013). Barriers to effective treatment of vaginal atrophy with local estrogen therapy. *International Journal of General Medicine,* 153-158. https://doi.org/10.2147/IJGM.S43192

Ritonja, J., Papantoniou, K., Ebenberger, A., Wagner, G., Gartlehner, G., Klerings, I., ... & Schernhammer, E. S. (2019). Effects of exposure to night shift work on cancer risk in workers. *The Cochrane Database of Systematic Reviews, 2019*(11), CD013466. doi:10.1002/14651858.CD013466

Sappenfeld et al. (2024, October*). National Survey of Children's Health.* HRSA Maternal and Child Health. https://mchb.hrsa.gov/sites/default/files/mchb/data-research/nsch-data-brief-adolescent-mental-behavioral-health-2023.pdf

Schug, T. T., Blawas, A. M., Gray, K., Heindel, J. J., & Lawler, C. P. (2015). Elucidating the links between endocrine disruptors and neurodevelopment. *Endocrinology, 156*(6), 1941-1951. https://doi.org/10.1210/en.2014-1734

SHRM. (2019). *The paralysis of depression in the workplace.* https://www.shrm.org/topics-tools/news/paralysis-depression-workplace

Silver. N. (n.d.). *Mood changes during perimenopause are real.* ACOG https://www.acog.org/womens-health/experts-and-stories/the-latest/mood-changes-during-perimenopause-are-real-heres-what-to-know

Spherical Insights. (2023, February). *Global bioidentical hormones market size, share, and COVID-19 impact analysis, by product (tablets & capsules, creams & gels, injectables, patches & implants, others), by administration (oral, parenteral), by end user (hospitals, clinics, others), by region (North America, Europe, Asia-Pacific, Latin America, Middle East, and Africa), Analysis and Forecast 2021 - 2030. Report ID: SI1537.* https://www.sphericalinsights.com/reports/bioidentical-hormones-market

The American Institute of Stress. (n.d.). *Workplace stress.* The American Institute of Stress. https://www.stress.org/workplace-stress/

The Carter Center. (2018). Mental illness will cost the world $16 USD trillion by 2030. *Psychiatric Times 35(11).* https://www.psychiatrictimes.com/view/mental-illness-will-cost-world-16-usd-trillion-2030

Traish, A. M., Miner, M. M., Morgentaler, A., & Zitzmann, M. (2011). Testosterone deficiency. *The American journal of medicine, 124*(7), 578-587. https://www.amjmed.com/article/s0002-9343(11)00274-9/fulltext#:~:text=Abstract,areas%20of%20concerns%20and%20uncertainty

Trasande, L. et al. (2015). Estimating burden and disease costs of exposure to endocrine-disrupting chemicals in the European Union. *Journal of Clinical Endocrinology & Metabolism.* https://doi.org/10.1210/jc.2014-4324

UC Berkeley School of Public Health. (n.d.). *HERMOSA study.* https://cerch.berkeley.edu/research-programs/hermosa-study

van Raalte, L. (2022, May 19). *4 significant physical benefits of hugging.* Psychology Today.

https://www.psychologytoday.com/us/blog/close-communication/202205/4-significant-physical-benefits-of-hugging

Vasconcelos, P., Carrito, M. L., Quinta-Gomes, A. L., Patrão, A. L., Nóbrega, C. A., Costa, P. A., & Nobre, P. J. (2024). Associations between sexual health and well-being: a systematic review. *Bulletin of the World Health Organization, 102*(12), 873.https://doi.org/10.2471/BLT.24.291565

Verified Market Reports. (Updated 2024, December). *Global menopause supplement market by type (tablets, capsules), by application (online pharmacies, retail pharmacies), by geographic scope and forecast report ID: 427744.* https://www.verifiedmarketreports.com/product/menopause-supplement-market/

Villines, Z. (2019). *What to know about sperm production.* Medical News Today. https://www.medicalnewstoday.com/articles/325906

Westervelt, A. (2015, April 30). Not so pretty: Women apply an average of 168 chemicals every day. *The Guardian.* https://www.theguardian.com/lifeandstyle/2015/apr/30/fda-cosmetics-health-nih-epa-environmental-working-group

Wikipedia. *Endometriosis.* https://en.wikipedia.org/wiki/Endometriosis

Wikipedia. *Premenstrual Syndrome.* https://en.wikipedia.org/wiki/Premenstrual_syndrome

World Health Organization. (2023). *Infertility prevalence estimates, 2023.* https://www.who.int/news/item/04-04-2023-1-in-6-people-globally-affected-by-infertility

World Health Organization. (2022). *Mental disorders.* https://www.who.int/news-room/fact-sheets/detail/mental-disorders

World Health Organization. (2016, April). *Investing in treatment for depression and anxiety leads to four-fold return.* https://www.who.int/news/item/13-04-2016-investing-in-treatment-for-depression-and-anxiety-leads-to-fourfold-return

World Health Organization. (2012). *State of the science of endocrine disrupting chemicals 2012.* https://www.who.int/publications/i/item/9789241505031

Zota, A. R., et al. (2016). Reducing phthalate, paraben, and phenol exposure from personal care products in adolescent girls: Findings from the HERMOSA Intervention Study. *Environmental Health Perspectives.* https://doi.org/10.1289/ehp.1510514

www.ingramcontent.com/pod-product-compliance
Lightning Source LLC
Chambersburg PA
CBHW070636030426
42337CB00020B/4039